Rational Therapeutics for Infants and Children

Workshop Summary

Sumner Yaffe, M.D., *Editor*

with the assistance of Ronald W. Estabrook,
Peter Bouxsein, Sarah Pitluck, and Jonathan R. Davis

Based on a Workshop of the
Roundtable on Research and Development of
Drugs, Biologics, and Medical Devices

Division of Health Sciences Policy

INSTITUTE OF MEDICINE

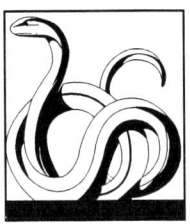

NATIONAL ACADEMY PRESS
Washington, DC

NATIONAL ACADEMY PRESS • 2101 Constitution Avenue, N.W. • Washington, D.C. 20418

NOTICE: The project that is the subject of this workshop summary was approved by the Governing Board of the National Research Council, whose members are drawn from the councils of the National Academy of Sciences, the National Academy of Engineering, and the Institute of Medicine. The members of the Roundtable responsible for the workshop summary were selected for their special competences and with regard for appropriate balance.

Support for this project was provided by the American Medical Association; Baxter International, Inc.; Eli Lilly; the U.S. Food and Drug Administration (Center for Biologics Evaluation and Research, Center for Devices and Radiological Health, and Center for Drug Evaluation and Research); the Health Industry Manufacturers Association; Hoffmann-La Roche; Merck & Co., Inc.; National Institutes of Health (Office of Rare Diseases and National Institute of Child Health and Human Development); Pfizer; and Wyeth-Ayerst. The views presented are those of the authors and are not necessarily those of the funding organizations.

This report is based on the proceedings of a workshop that was sponsored by the Roundtable on Research and Development of Drugs, Biologics, and Medical Devices. It is prepared in the form of a workshop summary by and in the name of the editor with the assistance of staff and consultants, as an individually authored document. Sections of the workshop summary not specifically attributed to an individual reflect the views of the editor and not those of the Roundtable on Research and Development of Drugs, Biologics, and Medical Devices. The content of those sections is based on the presentations and the discussions that took place during the workshop.

International Standard Book No. 0-309-06937-8

Additional copies of this workshop summary are available for sale from the National Academy Press, 2101 Constitution Avenue, N.W., Box 285, Washington, DC 20055. Call (800) 624-6242 or (202) 334-3313 (in the Washington metropolitan area), or visit the NAP's on-line bookstore at **www.nap.edu**.

For information about the Institute of Medicine, visit the IOM home page at **www.iom.edu**.

The full text of this Workshop Summary is available online at **www.nap.edu/readingroom**.

Copyright 2000 by the National Academy of Sciences. All rights reserved.

Printed in the United States of America.

The serpent has been a symbol of long life, healing, and knowledge among almost all cultures and religions since the beginning of recorded history. The image adopted as a logotype by the Institute of Medicine is based on a relief carving from ancient Greece, now held by the Staatliche Museen in Berlin.

THE NATIONAL ACADEMIES

National Academy of Sciences
National Academy of Engineering
Institute of Medicine
National Research Council

The **National Academy of Sciences** is a private, nonprofit, self-perpetuating society of distinguished scholars engaged in scientific and engineering research, dedicated to the furtherance of science and technology and to their use for the general welfare. Upon the authority of the charter granted to it by the Congress in 1863, the Academy has a mandate that requires it to advise the federal government on scientific and technical matters. Dr. Bruce M. Alberts is president of the National Academy of Sciences.

The **National Academy of Engineering** was established in 1964, under the charter of the National Academy of Sciences, as a parallel organization of outstanding engineers. It is autonomous in its administration and in the selection of its members, sharing with the National Academy of Sciences the responsibility for advising the federal government. The National Academy of Engineering also sponsors engineering programs aimed at meeting national needs, encourages education and research, and recognizes the superior achievements of engineers. Dr. William A. Wulf is president of the National Academy of Engineering.

The **Institute of Medicine** was established in 1970 by the National Academy of Sciences to secure the services of eminent members of appropriate professions in the examination of policy matters pertaining to the health of the public. The Institute acts under the responsibility given to the National Academy of Sciences by its congressional charter to be an adviser to the federal government and, upon its own initiative, to identify issues of medical care, research, and education. Dr. Kenneth I. Shine is president of the Institute of Medicine.

The **National Research Council** was organized by the National Academy of Sciences in 1916 to associate the broad community of science and technology with the Academy's purposes of furthering knowledge and advising the federal government. Functioning in accordance with general policies determined by the Academy, the Council has become the principal operating agency of both the National Academy of Sciences and the National Academy of Engineering in providing services to the government, the public, and the scientific and engineering communities. The Council is administered jointly by both Academies and the Institute of Medicine. Dr. Bruce M. Alberts and Dr. William A. Wulf are chairman and vice chairman, respectively, of the National Research Council.

ROUNDTABLE ON RESEARCH AND DEVELOPMENT OF DRUGS, BIOLOGICS, AND MEDICAL DEVICES

RONALD W. ESTABROOK (*Chair*), Virginia Lazenby O'Hara Professor of Biochemistry, University of Texas Southwestern Medical Center, Dallas

ARTHUR L. BEAUDET, Investigator, Howard Hughes Medical Institute, and Professor and Chair, Department of Molecular and Human Genetics, Baylor College of Medicine, Houston, (through February 1999)

LESLIE Z. BENET, Professor and Chair, Department of Biopharmaceutical Sciences, School of Pharmacy, University of California at San Francisco

D. BRUCE BURLINGTON, Director, Center for Devices and Radiological Health, U.S. Food and Drug Administration, Rockville, Maryland (through March 1999)

ROBERT CALIFF, Director, Duke Clinical Research Institute, Durham, North Carolina

MICHAEL D. CLAYMAN, Vice President, Global Regulatory Affairs, Lilly Research Laboratories, Indianapolis, Indiana

ADRIAN L. EDWARDS, Private Practice, Internal Medicine/Cardiology, The New York and Presbyterian Hospitals, New York City

DAVID W. FEIGAL, Director, Center for Devices and Radiological Health, U.S. Food and Drug Administration, Rockville, Maryland (from June 1999)

STEPHEN GROFT, Director, Office of Rare Diseases Research, National Institutes of Health, Bethesda, Maryland

ANNE B. JACKSON, American Association of Retired Persons, Washington, D.C.

ROBERT I. LEVY, Senior Vice President, Science and Technology, American Home Products, Wyeth-Ayerst Research, Madison, New Jersey

MICHAEL R. McGARVEY, Chief Medical Officer, Blue Cross and Blue Shield of New Jersey, Inc., Newark

KSHITIJ MOHAN, Corporate Vice President for Research and Technical Services, Baxter Health Care Corporation, Roundlake, Illinois

STUART L. NIGHTINGALE, Associate Commissioner, Health Affairs, Food and Drug Administration, Rockville, Maryland

PAUL GRANT ROGERS, Partner, Hogan & Hartson, Washington, D.C.

DANIEL SECKINGER, Group Vice President, Professional Standards, American Medical Association, Chicago (through December 1997)

WHAIJEN SOO, Vice President, Clinical Sciences, Roche Pharmaceuticals, Hoffmann-La Roche, Inc., Nutley, New Jersey

REED TUCKSON, Senior Vice President, Professional Standards, American Medical Association, Chicago (from October 1998)

JANET WOODCOCK, Director, Center for Drug Evaluation and Research, U.S. Food and Drug Administration, Rockville, Maryland

SUMNER YAFFE, Director, Center for Research for Mothers and Children, National Institute of Child Health and Human Development, National Institutes of Health, Bethesda, Maryland

KATHRYN ZOON, Director, Center for Biologics Evaluation and Research, U.S. Food and Drug Administration, Rockville, Maryland

Liaisons to the Roundtable

JAMES S. BENSON, Executive Vice President, Technology and Regulatory Affairs, Health Industry Manufacturers Association, Washington, D.C.

C. THOMAS CASKEY, Senior Vice President for Research, Merck & Co., Inc., West Point, Pennsylvania

BRIAN J. MALKIN, Associate Director for Patents and Hearings, Office of Health Affairs, U.S. Food and Drug Administration, Rockville, Maryland

BERT SPILKER, Senior Vice President, Scientific and Regulatory Affairs, Pharmaceutical Research and Manufacturers of America, Washington, D.C.

Study Staff

JONATHAN R. DAVIS, Senior Program Officer
PETER BOUXSEIN, Senior Program Officer
SARAH PITLUCK, Research Assistant
VIVIAN P. NOLAN, Research Associate
NICOLE AMADO, Project Assistant (until August 1999)

Division Staff

ANDREW M. POPE, Division Director
ALDEN CHANG, Project Assistant
THELMA COX, Project Assistant
SETH KELLY, Project Assistant
CARLOS GABRIEL, Financial Associate
HALLIE WILFERT, Administrative Assistant

Consultant

KATHI HANNA

Copy Editor

MICHAEL HAYES

REVIEWERS

All presenters at the workshop have reviewed and approved their respective sections of this workshop summary for accuracy. In addition, this workshop summary has been reviewed in draft form by independent reviewers chosen for their diverse perspectives and technical expertise, in accordance with procedures approved by the National Research Council's Report Review Committee. The purpose of this independent review is to provide candid and critical comments that will assist the Institute of Medicine (IOM) in making the published workshop summary as sound as possible and to ensure that the workshop summary meets institutional standards. The review comments and draft manuscript remain confidential to protect the integrity of the deliberative process.

Although the independent reviewers have provided many constructive comments and suggestions, responsibility for the final content of this workshop summary rests solely with the IOM. The Roundtable and IOM thank the following individuals for their participation in the review process:

Cheston M. Berlin, University Professor of Pediatrics and Professor of Pharmacology, Department of Pediatrics, Milton S. Hershey Medical Center, Hershey, Pennsylvania

Jeffrey L. Blumer, Professor of Pediatrics and Pharmacology, Case Western Reserve University and Chief, Division of Pediatric Pharmacology and Critical Care, Rainbow Babies and Children's Hospital, Cleveland

Sanford N. Cohen, Cape Coral, Florida

Ronald N. Hines, Codirector, Birth Defects Research Center, and Professor of Pediatrics and Pharmacology/Toxicology, Department of Pediatrics, Medical College of Wisconsin and Children's Hospital of Wisconsin, Milwaukee

Frank L. Hurley, Chief Scientific Officer, Quintiles Transnational Corporation, Arlington, Virginia

Gideon Koren, Member, American Board of Medical Toxicology and Fellow Royal College of Physicians and Surgeons

Allan M. Korn, Senior Vice President of Clinical Affairs and Chief Medical Officer, Blue Cross and Blue Shield Association, Chicago

Allen A. Mitchell, Director, Sloan Epidemiology Unit, Professor of Epidemiology and Pediatrics, Boston University School of Public Health and Medicine, Brookline

Robert M. Ward, Professor, Pediatrics and Director, Pediatric Pharmacology Program, Division of Neonatology, University of Utah, Salt Lake City

Mel Worth, Scholar-in-Residence, Institute of Medicine, The National Academies, Washington, D.C.

Preface

The Institute of Medicine's (IOM's) Roundtable on Research and Development of Drugs, Biologics, and Medical Devices evolved from the Forum on Drug Development, which was established in 1986. Sponsor representatives and IOM determined the importance of maintaining a neutral setting for discussions regarding long-term and politically sensitive issues justified the need to revise and enhance past efforts. The new Roundtable is intended to be a mechanism by which a broad group of experts from the public[*] and private sectors can be convened to conduct a dialogue and exchange information related to the development of drugs, biologics, and medical devices. Members have expertise in clinical medicine, pediatrics, clinical pharmacology, health policy, health insurance, industrial management, and product development; and they represent interests that address all facets of public policy issues.

From time to time, the Roundtable requests that a workshop be conducted for the purpose of exploring a specific topic in detail and obtaining the views of additional experts. Summaries of these workshops are prepared and disseminated to make the discussion readily accessible to the members of the Roundtable and other interested parties. Such workshop summaries are intended only to convey the presentations and discussion that took place at the workshop; they do not include any conclusions or recommendations on the part of the Roundtable or any further data or analysis of the issues.

---

[*]Representatives of federal agencies serve in an ex officio capacity. An ex officio member of a group is one who is a member automatically by virtue of holding a particular office or membership in another body.

The first workshop for the Roundtable was held on April 14 and 15, 1998, and was entitled Assuring Data Quality and Validity in Clinical Trials for Regulatory Decision Making. The summary on that workshop is available from IOM.

This workshop summary covers the second workshop, which was held on May 24 and 25, 1999, and which was aimed at facilitating the development and proper use of drugs, biologics, and medical devices for infants and children. It explores the scientific underpinnings and clinical needs, as well as the regulatory, legal, and ethical issues, raised by this area of research and development.

The environment for pediatric therapeutics has been altered by two important developments. First, the Food and Drug Administration Modernization Act, enacted in 1997, provides incentives to pharmaceutical manufacturers that conduct acceptable studies with children and drugs identified by the U.S. Food and Drug Administration, to be ones for which information on the effects on the pediatric population would be beneficial. Second, in December 1998 the U.S. Food and Drug Administration published a final rule that established certain requirements for studies with the pediatric population and drugs that significantly affect infants and children.

This workshop addressed many important issues. For example, many questions about the biochemistry of the enzymes involved in drug metabolism remain unanswered, in particular, the variability in the responses of individuals to drugs. The differences in the pharmacodynamics and pharmacogenetics of drug metabolism between children and adults remain undetermined. In addition, the influence of diet on the process of induction of these enzymes during the various stages of development deserves extensive study. Three sets of concerns need to be addressed to advance the development of rational therapeutics for infants and children:

1. What is the scientific basis for differences in the responses to drugs of humans during their life spans, from the time of development in fetuses, infants, and young children through the process of aging?
2. How do the metabolic, immune, and other systems of infants and children function differently at various stages of growth, what are the factors that influence these differences, and do they alter responses to drugs?
3. What data need to be known to determine pediatric drug dosages? Can dosages be extrapolated from data for adults? How can responses to drugs be evaluated ethically in children?

This summary on the workshop is organized as topic-by-topic descriptions of the presentations and discussions that occurred during the workshop. Although the proceedings were rich and wide-ranging, this workshop summary does not purport to be a comprehensive or exhaustive exploration of the issues discussed. Nor does it represent a consensus of views or opinions from IOM or the Roundtable. Rather, it summarizes a dialogue among representatives from

PREFACE

different sectors and their thoughts on what research and what public policy issues may merit further attention. The editor's summary material at the beginning of each section provides some context and overview of the identified presentations.

On behalf of the members of the Roundtable, I express my warmest appreciation to the authors of this workshop summary for providing a timely and useful summary of the issues raised and the discussions that occurred. I also want to thank the individuals and organizations that gave valuable time to provide information and insight to the Roundtable through participation in the workshop. Each of the following contributed greatly: Charles H. Ballow, Kaleida Health Millard Fillmore Hospital; Mark Batshaw, George Washington University Medical Center, Children's Research Institute, Children's National Medical Center; Emmett Clemente, Ascent Pediatrics, Inc.; Thierry Cresteil, Centre National de la Recherche Scientifique, Institut Gustave Roussy, Villejuif, France; Sherin U. Devaskar, Magee Women's Hospital, University of Pittsburgh School of Medicine; Susan Ellenberg, Center for Biologics Evaluation and Research, U.S. Food and Drug Administration; David Feigal, Jr., Center for Devices and Radiological Health, U.S. Food and Drug Administration; Jane Henney, U.S. Food and Drug Administration; Ralph Kauffman, Children's Mercy Hospital; Greg Kearns, Division of Pediatric Clinical Pharmacology, Children's Mercy Hospital; Michael Labson, Covington & Burling; Steve Leeder, Children's Mercy Hospital; Murray Lumpkin, Center for Drug Evaluation and Research, U.S. Food and Drug Administration; Michael McGarvey, Blue Cross and Blue Shield of New Jersey, Inc.; Dianne Murphy, Center for Drug Evaluation and Research, U.S. Food and Drug Administration; Robert M. (Skip) Nelson, Medical College of Wisconsin; David Poplack, Baylor College of Medicine and Texas Children's Cancer Center; Stephen Spielberg, R.W. Johnson Pharmaceutical Research Institute; Stanley J. Szefler, National Jewish Medical and Research Center, University of Colorado Health Sciences Center; Robert Temple, Center for Drug Evaluation and Research, U.S. Food and Drug Administration; John Watchko, Department of Pediatrics, Magee Women's Hospital, University of Pittsburgh School of Medicine; Karen Weiss, Center for Biologics Evaluation and Research, U.S. Food and Drug Administration; and John T. Wilson, Department of Pediatrics, Louisiana State University Medical Center.

I also thank the following IOM staff for their valuable contributions in this activity: Vivian Nolan, Nicole Amado, Alden Chang, and Thelma Cox. Consultant and technical writer Kathi Hanna contributed significantly to the writing of many sections of the workshop summary. The extensive commentary and suggestions made by the copy editor, Michael Hayes, are gratefully acknowledged.

Finally, the Roundtable and IOM also wish to thank the sponsors that supported this activity. Financial support for this project was provided by the

American Medical Association, Baxter International Inc., Eli Lilly, U.S. Food and Drug Administration (Center for Biologics Evaluation and Research, Center for Devices and Radiological Health, and Center for Drug Evaluation and Research), the Health Industry Manufacturers Association, Hoffmann-La Roche, Merck & Co., Inc., National Institutes of Health (Office of Rare Diseases and National Institute of Child Health and Human Development), Pfizer, and Wyeth-Ayerst.

Sumner Yaffe, M.D.
Editor

Contents

EDITOR'S SUMMARY 1

1 INTRODUCTION 8
   Science, Challenges, and Children, 8
   First Steps, 8
   New Rule Making, 10
   Challenges to Studies with Children, 11
   The Role of FDA, 12

2 SIMILARITIES AND DISSIMILARITIES IN PHYSIOLOGY,
   METABOLISM, AND DISEASE STATES AND RESPONSES
   TO THERAPY IN CHILDREN AND ADULTS 14
   Historical Background, 15
   Differences Between Children and Adults, 16
   Differential Responses of Children to Drugs, 21
   Molecular Basis of Drug Metabolism, 23
   Gene Expression and Ontogeny of Drug Metabolism, 29

3 PHARMACOKINETICS AND PHARMACODYNAMICS IN
   CHILDREN VERSUS ADULTS 34
   Drug Metabolism in Children and Adolescents: Insights from
      Therapeutic Adventures, 35
   Ontogeny of P-Glycoprotein, an ATP-Dependent Transmembrane
      Efflux Pump, 41

Developmental Aspects of Glucose Transporters, 44
Formulation, 46
Anti-Infectives, 48
Childhood Asthma, 50
Pediatric Oncology, 58

**4 EXTRAPOLATION OF SAFETY AND EFFICACY
DATA TO CHILDREN** 61
Special Considerations for Evaluating Medical Devices in Infants
and Children, 62
Defining Surrogate Endpoints and Biomarkers for Drug Action in
Trials with Pediatric Subjects, 64
Prediction of Long-Term Effects on Postnatal Brain Development, 66
Evaluating Biologic Therapeutics in Pediatric Clinical Trials, 68

**5 RAISING AWARENESS OF REGULATORY, LEGAL,
AND ETHICAL ISSUES** 71
FDA Perspective on New Regulations, 72
Roles of Institutional Review Boards and Data-Monitoring
Committees in Clinical Trials, 73
Ethics of Drug and Biologic Research in Infants and Children, 76
Legal and Regulatory Considerations for the Conduct of
Clinical Trials with Pediatric Populations, 85
International Development of Drugs for Pediatric Patients: An
Industry Perspective, 88
Panel Discussion, 90

6 CONCLUDING REMARKS 92

REFERENCES 95

APPENDIXES
A Workshop Agenda, 105
B Biographies, 111

Editor's Summary

Sumner Yaffe, M.D., *Editor*

The development of rational therapeutics for infants and children has recently received much attention from the academic community, industry, the U.S. Congress, and the federal government. The members of the Roundtable on Research and Development of Drugs, Biologics, and Medical Devices recognized that a variety of interesting and challenging issues are being raised, from several different perspectives, among a diverse group of interested and affected parties. Consequently, they requested that a workshop be held to explore such issues in depth. This report summarizes the proceedings of that workshop.

The U.S. Food and Drug Administration (FDA), the federal regulatory body involved during the development, preclinical studies, and clinical trial phases of new drug discovery and testing with humans, requires that companies provide evidence of the safety and effectiveness of a product before marketing of that product. The protocols used to meet this requirement have been in effect for the last three decades and have historically been primarily confined to studies with adult populations. For many years, however, it was considered to be unethical to enroll children in clinical studies.

However, over time it became increasingly recognized that children are not small adults and that special considerations for this population are critical. In 1977, the American Academy of Pediatrics declared that it was unethical to ex-

---

The content of this summary reflects the views of the editor, which are not those of the Roundtable. It is based solely on the presentations and the discussions that took place during the workshop.

pect physicians to prescribe therapeutic agents to children in the absence of specific evidence on how children responded to such agents; to do so amounted to conducting an uncontrolled experiment when dispensing a prescription to a child. FDA regulations published in 1994, 1997, and 1998 significantly changed the circumstances under which therapeutics are prescribed for pediatric patients. Manufacturers, for example, are now required to evaluate the safety and effectiveness of certain new and marketed drugs and biologic products in pediatric patients. In addition, the Food and Drug Administration Modernization Act, enacted in 1997, provides a financial incentive, in the form of a 6-month extension of patent exclusivity, for manufacturers to undertake studies on the safety and efficacy of drugs prescribed for children.

Thus, through the regulatory process, financial incentives are now provided to pharmaceutical sponsors who investigate drugs and biologics in children and who present such information in their new drug application submissions. However, the exact relationship among these provisions remains to be determined. Although the main directions for undertaking the requisite studies on the proper use of therapeutics in children are in place, many challenges and issues remain. The term *pediatric population*, for instance, does not encompass one homogeneous group of patients; instead, it consists of a collection of highly variable subgroups, from neonates, to infants, to teenagers. Recruitment of subjects for a clinical trial is another challenge that involves complicated issues of informed consent of children and parents. Another critical variable in this equation involves consideration of the growth and developmental changes that occur through infancy, childhood, and adolescence, which in turn complicates determination of appropriate surrogate endpoints and drug dosages. Completing clinical trials in children is yet another challenge, given the required long-term follow-up studies.

Although the regulatory process encourages pharmaceutical sponsors to investigate drugs and biologics in studies with children and rewards them for doing so, until now the primary emphasis has been on the collection of data concerning drug kinetics and, to a lesser extent, dynamics in pediatric and aged individuals. Little emphasis has been placed on understanding the mechanistic basis for the differences and the similarities that are observed. Consequently, there is a dearth of information on the basic mechanisms responsible for the pharmacokinetic and pharmacodynamic behaviors of major classes of drugs in these special populations. Although maturation is one area of investigation known to influence drug disposition in children, information on other processes, such as ontogeny of drug biotransformation pathways, drug transport systems, and pharmacologic receptor functions and their regulation and gene expression, is generally lacking or is at best rudimentary.

Advances in molecular biology have resulted in an unprecedented surge in the number of new therapeutic agents available for testing in studies with children. There is a concern, however, that a shortage of trained clinical pharmacologists (particularly those who can integrate the field of molecular biology with clinical investigation), the increasing number of drugs available for testing, and the limited capacity to conduct clinical trials with children may still result in the prescription of too many drugs for children in the absence of good evidence for their safety and efficacy in that population. Additionally, on the basis of a lack of experience, there are concerns about the new FDA regulations that permit a drug to be prescribed for a pediatric patient on the basis of adequate and well-controlled studies with adults if the course of the disease and the effects of the drug are sufficiently similar in the pediatric and adult populations. Comparison of the pediatric and adult populations needs to take several factors into account, including pathophysiology and natural history of diseases common to both groups and the host reactions to disease and therapeutic agents (including pharmacodynamics and toxic reactions).

The workshop summarized in this report explored how scientists in industry, academia, and the government can develop a research strategy to gather the needed information to facilitate the development process for therapeutic drugs and biologics designed for use in the pediatric population. The workshop focused on four major areas of importance for improving understanding of the development and testing of drugs and biologics in studies with pediatric populations, as well as facilitating future planning in this area:

- how children are similar or dissimilar to adults with regard to physiology, drug metabolism, immunology, cognitive effects, and response to disease states and therapy;
- the identification of new advances in biomedical science that are uniquely applicable to children and that could be applied to the development and testing of drugs and biologics in studies with children;
- the special requirements in evaluating drugs and biologics in studies with pediatric populations, including an assessment of when and how safety and efficacy data can be used for children; and
- an examination of the many legal and regulatory issues in evaluating new drugs and biologics in studies with pediatric populations, as well as interrelated social and ethical concerns.

The following sections highlight major themes discussed in the workshop presentations.

SIMILARITIES AND DISSIMILARITIES IN PHYSIOLOGY, METABOLISM, AND DISEASE STATES AND RESPONSES TO THERAPY IN CHILDREN AND ADULTS

The pediatric population often responds to drugs and biologics differently than adults do. Generally, the drug prescription guidelines that practitioners use have not always been based on biologic or pharmacologic principles when they extrapolate the drug doses used for adults to infants and children. Not only have the guidelines tended to be simplistic, in that they assume a linear relationship between children and adults, but they have also not made allowances for the complex changes in growth and development that take place during childhood. A number of quantitative and qualitative differences in the anatomy and physiology of the infant and developing child can affect the absorption, distribution, metabolism, and excretion of various drugs and other xenobiotic compounds. Additionally, children differ from adults not only in anatomical and physiological ways but also in the types of diseases from which they suffer and in their manifestations of these diseases that they do have in common with adults. These factors can determine the types of therapies developed for children as well as the design of studies that evaluate new therapeutic agents.

Adverse experiences to drugs that have been tolerated by adults have been observed in children when the drugs have not been adequately studied before their use in the pediatric population. A structured analysis of children's responses to drugs that are tolerated by adults could strengthen the safety component of the study design. The ontogeny of drug-metabolizing enzymes in humans, for instance, may explain several differences in the responses to drugs by adult and pediatric populations. Understanding the relative role of absorption in drug biotransformation may also lead to better understanding of the drug-metabolizing abilities of the different populations. Phenotyping studies of drug biotransformation could also help explain differential responses to drugs.

The results of studies with adults may not always be extrapolated to children because growth and development issues add a range of complicated variables to the already intricate realm of drug metabolism and pharmacodynamics. Studies of drugs for use in children must be designed to account for the complex developmental changes that can affect drug biodisposition and pharmacodynamics.

PHARMACOKINETICS AND PHARMACODYNAMICS IN CHILDREN VERSUS ADULTS

Pharmacokinetics and pharmacodynamics are very different in children and adults. The pharmacokinetics of many drugs vary with age (Kearns, 1998). For instance, because of the rapid changes in size, body composition, and organ function that occur during the first year of life, clinicians as well as pharmacokineticists and toxicologists are presented with challenges in prescribing safe and effective doses of therapeutic agents (Milsap and Jusko, 1994). Studies with adolescents reveal even more complexity in drug metabolism and differences in drug metabolism between the sexes.

The therapeutic value of understanding differences in pharmacokinetics because of developmental factors thus relies on an ability to understand better the dose versus concentration versus effect profile for a specific drug in patients of various ages (Kearns, 1998). In turn, recognition of differences in pharmacokinetics because of developmental factors can be invaluable for interpretation of data and improving and guiding the design of clinical trials on drug disposition and efficacy.

EXTRAPOLATION OF SAFETY AND EFFICACY DATA TO CHILDREN

Extrapolation to children of safety and efficacy data generated for adults requires careful attention to potentially important differences between these two populations. The safety of drugs, for instance, needs to be supported by appropriate research with the targeted age group. Some medications that are completely safe for adults may produce toxic effects in children. An assessment of pharmacokinetic-pharmacodynamic relationships, however, by use of a surrogate and comparison of those results with those for adults may suffice as a basis for approval of the drug for use in the pediatric population or help determine the doses to be used in clinical trial.

Unlike drugs, the majority of which are for oral administration, the majority of therapeutic biologics are for parenteral use only. Thus, many of the formulation issues for biologics to be used in the pediatric population are similar to the formulation issues for parenteral drugs to be used in the adult population. Because of their distinctive properties, the use of biologics results in unique safety concerns that require different types of monitoring, such as for adventitious agents that occur as a result of treatment with the biologic, or for reactogenicity. There is some concern about therapeutic biologics because little is known about the long-term effects of treatment with such agents, especially their effects on developing children. Many questions about the evaluation of biologics in the pediatric population need to be addressed; no simple approach is available.

The requirements for the safety and efficacy of medical devices are different from those for the safety and efficacy of drugs and biologics. Not only can the size of a device pose engineering problems, but also hormonal influences and the activity levels of patients need to be factored into the design of devices. Obtaining approval for use of a device in the pediatric population is also not an easy undertaking; ample evidence indicating that it has been properly designed for children and that the safety and efficacy are demonstrated rather than presumed must be made available.

RAISING AWARENESS OF REGULATORY, LEGAL, AND ETHICAL ISSUES

Every year, information necessary for the proper use of drugs and biologics in infants and children is lacking for more than half of newly approved drugs and biologics that are likely to be used by children. This is often because children are not sufficiently included in research studies. Pediatric clinical trials involve many logistical challenges as well as legal and regulatory considerations. For instance, a special consideration is informed consent and whether parental consent, the assent of the child, or both are required.

FDA's new Pediatric Rule makes it more likely that children will receive improved treatment, because physicians will have more complete information on how drugs affect children and the appropriate doses for each age group (FDA, 1998e). The rule also allows FDA to require industry to test already marketed products in studies with pediatric populations in certain compelling circumstances, such as when a drug is commonly prescribed for use in children and the absence of adequate testing and labeling could pose significant risks.

OPPORTUNITIES FOR IMPROVING THE PROCESS

To conduct the necessary studies of drugs with pediatric populations, adequate numbers of patients and researchers are needed. New laboratory methodologies need to be developed to make drug testing more applicable to children. It will be important to address the lack of appropriate formulations and commercial incentives for some drugs that are important for the pediatric population.

Recent efforts to grant exclusivity to sponsors of pediatric drugs are aimed at achieving a societal good. It has been a tool previously used by the U.S. Congress to promote the development of orphan and generic drugs. Now, the Congress is again using this tool to encourage the development of drugs for use in infants and children.

This financial incentive carries with it a serious scientific responsibility. It is likely to result in changes in attitudes about the feasibility of studies with children and, as a result, a larger infrastructure for studying drugs in children. Hopefully, this will result in better drug labeling for the pediatric population, more appropriate formulations, better dosing guidelines for more age ranges, and better information about efficacy and toxicity.

It will be important to carefully evaluate, over the next several years, how well this financial incentive achieved its stated objectives. Doing so poses several challenges:

- Industry, government, and academia must together develop some good metrics to determine if the goals of the new incentive programs have been met.
- If heavy reliance is placed on extrapolation of data for adult populations, there must be a way of evaluating, over the long term, whether it is working well.
- A means of long-term monitoring must be developed, financed, and conducted to assess the effects of drugs on children's growth and their neuronal, psychosocial, and endocrinologic maturation.

If it is concluded that this incentive program does work for the pediatric population and is worth the cost, it may encourage its application to other populations, such as pregnant women, elderly people, or minority groups. If it is applicable to these other groups, will it be at the expense of maintaining the program for children?

1

Introduction

SCIENCE, CHALLENGES, AND CHILDREN

Presented by Jane Henney, M.D.
Commissioner, U.S. Food and Drug Administration

During recent years, the development of rational therapeutics for infants and children has received a great deal of attention from the academic community, the U.S. Congress, industry, and the federal government, particularly the U.S. Food and Drug Administration (FDA). Although FDA has been in existence for nearly 100 years, it had limited authority with respect to regulating drugs until the 1930s. During that time, however, it was charged with overseeing the evaluation of drug safety. It was not until the 1960s that FDA gained the regulatory authority to require companies to provide evidence that a product was effective before marketing of the product.

For the next three decades, demonstration of safety and effectiveness was largely confined to studies in adult populations. Children were not usually entered into clinical studies, with the exception of those for the development of vaccines, because it was considered unethical to enroll them in experiments. Although physicians and parents wanted adequate use information for products given to sick children, they feared that studies conducted with such children would be deleterious and perhaps unacceptable. These concerns still linger, although perhaps differently so for the parents of children affected by serious or life-threatening diseases and illnesses. Industry was also reluctant to study children because of concerns about liability and because of the large investments in drugs for potentially small markets.

FIRST STEPS

In 1977, the American Academy of Pediatrics made a first move to change the status quo. The Academy asserted that it was unethical to adhere to a system that forces physicians to use therapeutic agents in essentially uncontrolled experiments every time that they write a prescription for a child. Furthermore, the Academy stated that it was imperative that new drugs intended for use in children be studied in children under controlled circumstances so that the benefits of therapeutic advances could become available to all who need them.

These principles made a powerful, yet simple statement: children deserve and should have the same standard as adults when it comes to therapeutics. If adequate and well-controlled studies are needed to determine the efficacy of products used for adults, then the same should be true for products used for children. This statement of principle shifted everyone's thinking about clinical testing of medical products in the pediatric population. No longer were the experts focused on the dogma of how unethical it was to study the effects of drugs in children. It became unethical not to conduct such studies.

In 1979, FDA confirmed the need to have information on how best to use a product in the pediatric population by issuing regulations. The position of the agency was that if statements were to be made regarding pediatric use of a drug for an indication approved for adults, such statements were required to be based on substantial evidence derived from adequate and well-controlled studies, unless the requirement was waived.

Unfortunately, this particular regulation did not generate the intended response. Few clinical trials with the pediatric population were initiated. The regulation did not provide incentives for companies to conduct such studies, nor were there repercussions for not doing so. Thus, for two-thirds to three-quarters of all drugs used by the pediatric population, directions for use by children that were based on data from clinical trials were not available.

More than a decade passed before the agency took a more assertive stance. In 1994, FDA issued a final rule requiring drug manufacturers to survey existing data and determine whether those data were sufficient to support the presentation of additional pediatric use information in a drug's labeling. The rule explicitly recognized that controlled clinical studies conducted to support pediatric use need not be carried out with a pediatric population if the course of the disease and the effects of the drug are sufficiently similar in children and adults. Extrapolation of adult effectiveness data to pediatric patients was permitted. In these cases, controlled clinical studies with adults, together with other information such as pharmacokinetics and adverse reaction data for pediatric patients, could be found to be sufficient to establish the safety and effectiveness of a drug in children.

Under the 1994 rule, if a manufacturer determined that existing data permitted modification of the label's pediatric use information, the manufacturer had to submit a supplemental new drug application to FDA to seek approval of these labeling changes. It is important to recognize that this rule did not impose a general requirement that manufacturers carry out studies if existing information was not sufficient to support pediatric use information. Instead, where there was insufficient information to support a pediatric indication or pediatric use statement, the rule allowed the manufacturer instead to include a statement in the drug's labeling which clarified that: "Safety and effectiveness in pediatric patients have not been established."

More than half of the responses to the rule used the latter approach. Approximately 75 percent of the applications submitted did not show significant improvement in pediatric use information. The actions taken by FDA produced some gains in labeling for pediatric use, but did not substantially increase the number of drugs and biologic products for which there was adequate pediatric use information.

Indeed, when the agency compared the number of new molecular entities approved in 1991 and 1996 with their potential usefulness in pediatric patients—using a specific process to assess the adequacy of labeling of those drugs for pediatric use—56 percent of the products approved in 1991 had some labeling for pediatric use at the time of approval. Yet in 1996 this number had fallen to only 37 percent. Of the seven new molecular entities that were approved in 1991 and for which postapproval pediatric studies were promised, only one had pediatric use labeling by 1997. Clearly, if the goal of ensuring the safety and effectiveness of drugs and biologic products for pediatric patients was to be met, additional steps needed to be taken.

NEW RULE MAKING

In August 1997, FDA proposed a rule with provisions that required the manufacturers of certain new and marketed drugs and biologic products to evaluate the safety and effectiveness of their products in pediatric patients. This included new drugs or biologic products that would provide a meaningful therapeutic benefit to pediatric patients over existing treatments, or that were likely to be used by a substantial number of pediatric patients. The proposed regulation also included certain marketed drugs or biologic products, such as those indicated for a very significant or life-threatening illness.

In the preamble to the proposed rule, the agency noted that financial and other incentives to manufacturers, although largely beyond FDA's authority at that time, could further increase the number of drugs and biologics with adequate labeling for pediatric use. The incentive approach was provided by Congress in the Food and Drug Administration Modernization Act of 1997. The legislation includes "Section III," or the pediatric exclusivity provision. This provision created a financial incentive—an additional 6 months of market exclusivity to industry—for conducting studies of new drugs as well as drugs that were already on the market and for which the patent was still intact in the pediatric population (FDA, 1997b).

FDA also initiated other actions to encourage the development of adequate pediatric use information. These included publication of guidance on clinical trial designs for the assessment of pediatric pharmacokinetics of drug and biologic products, development of an initial guidance document on clinical trials with pediatric subjects, and discussions with the pharmaceutical industry on a policy exempting user fees for pediatric supplements.

In late 1998, FDA finalized its previously proposed regulations regarding studies in pediatric populations. Although no products found to be safe and effective in adults are to be—or have been—delayed or denied approval because of a lack of testing in the pediatric population, there is now a requirement for a manufacturer to conduct trials with children in an expeditious manner.

The final rule and the pediatric exclusivity provisions are critical to ensuring needed and timely development of drugs for use by the pediatric population. From November 1997 to May 1999, FDA witnessed more interest and activity in this field than in the past several decades. Between June 1998 and May 1999, FDA received more than 115 proposals from sponsors requesting permission to perform various studies with pediatric populations. In comparison, there were 70 commitments for Phase 4 studies with pediatric subjects made from 1991 to 1997.

CHALLENGES TO STUDIES WITH CHILDREN

Since the new rule has been in effect, FDA has observed a needed shift in attitude toward clinical testing in pediatric populations on the part of all involved: the agency, industry, researchers, and parents. However, challenges remain.

First, the term *pediatric population* does not refer to a homogeneous group of patients but really refers to a collection of highly variable subgroups from neonates, to infants, to teenagers. Neonates are often seen as one of the most difficult age groups to test because of the potential differences in how their bodies will metabolize *and respond to* a given drug. However, that group has the advantage of being highly monitored by a variety of devices and of being under the care of highly skilled hospital staff. Infants, on the other hand, do not receive the 24-hour monitoring given to neonates. If they do, it is often provided by their parents, who are not always the most unbiased observers. On the other end of the spectrum are adolescents. Although unlike the neonate or the infant, adolescents are able to communicate with providers and parents, they might not always be willing to do so.

Recruitment of subjects for a clinical trial is also a challenge. It requires individuals who can understand parental concerns and communicate that understanding. Often, a number of family members need to be involved in this decision-making activity. An investigator's ability to repeatedly explain the study to parents, grandparents, and other significant family members can be critical to a trial's success.

Defining what benefit a child may derive from the additional discomforts of blood drawing, frequent hospital or clinic visits, or other inconveniences that the child may experience is an important aspect of ensuring the ethical implementation of such a study. Trial design issues, such as the requirement for hospitalization, the duration of a study, the number and timing of the evaluation visits, and the need to decrease or stop current therapy to initiate study therapy are all challenges that make study recruitment for the pediatric population different from that for the adult population. The parent, caretaker, or older child must weigh the benefits of the study to the patient or themselves versus the costs of the loss of work or school and the disruption to the family and daily living that may result from participation in a study.

Another critical variable that must be considered for children involves growth and maturation and the expected changes that occur throughout infancy, childhood, and adolescence. It is difficult to define the effects of chronic therapy on children and to differentiate their positive effects or possible negative effects on the dynamic processes of childhood.

Long-term follow-up over several years after the receipt of therapeutic interventions may be needed to assess neural development, behavior, and bone and joint growth. Another challenge that is simple in studies with adults but that is complex in studies with pediatric populations is determination of appropriate endpoints. Fundamental measurements, such as vital signs, height, and weight are dynamic measurements for children. Thus, outcome measures must be modified. For example, for children the important outcome measure is the rate of weight gain, not simply weight maintenance or weight gain, as it would be for adults.

Another example is pain scales, which in studies with adults are represented by a bar with numerical options extending from one extreme to the other. The study subject selects his or her level of pain (e.g., 3 on a scale of 10). This concept is often not transferable as ordinal numbers to children; thus, a pain scale that depicts sad and happy faces is sometimes used in an attempt to capture the same endpoint measurement.

Cost is also a challenge involved with completing clinical trials with children. Enrollment of children in clinical trials often requires long-term follow-up, which requires expertise, technology, and personnel, all of which are expensive. In addition, research is needed to assist those who conduct clinical trials with children to provide them with the technology and methods that allow studies to be conducted where it was not possible before. For example, innovations in such areas as blood sampling and diagnostic techniques are needed.

THE ROLE OF FDA

The days of reluctance to conduct clinical testing of new drugs in the pediatric population are past. FDA has the important task of defining what studies in pediatric populations are needed and requesting or requiring sponsors to perform such studies. The agency is committed to working with the scientific, professional, and consumer communities to improve this area of research and thus enhance the health of children.

2
Similarities and Dissimilarities in Physiology, Metabolism, and Disease States and Responses to Therapy in Children and Adults

The pediatric population often responds to drugs and other therapeutics differently than adults do. Generally, the guidelines that practitioners use when they prescribe drugs have not been based on biologic or pharmacologic principles when they extrapolate the drug doses used for adults to infants and children. Not only have the guidelines tended to be simplistic in that they assume a linear relationship between children and adults, but they have also not made allowances for the complex changes in growth and development that take place during childhood. A number of quantitative and qualitative differences in the anatomy and physiology of the infant and developing child can affect the absorption, distribution, metabolism, and excretion of various drugs and other xenobiotic compounds. Additionally, children differ from adults not only in anatomical and physiological ways but also in the types of diseases from which they suffer and in the manifestations of those diseases that they do have in common with adults. These factors can determine the types of therapies developed for children as well as the design of studies that evaluate new therapeutic agents.

Adverse experiences to drugs that have been tolerated by adults have been observed in children when the drugs have not been adequately studied before their use in the pediatric population. A structured analysis of children's responses to drugs that are tolerated by adults could strengthen the safety component of the study design. The ontogeny of drug-metabolizing enzymes in humans, for instance, may explain several differences in the responses to drugs by adult and pediatric populations. Understanding the relative role of absorption in drug biotransformation may also lead to better understanding of the drug-metabolizing abilities of the different populations. Phenotyping studies of drug biotransformation could also help explain differential responses to drugs.

The results of studies with adults thus cannot typically be extrapolated to children because growth and development issues add a range of complicated variables to the already intricate realm of drug metabolism and pharmacodynamics. Studies of drugs for use in children must be designed to account for the complex developmental changes that can affect drug biodisposition and pharmacodynamics. The following summaries of the presentations at the workshop examine the uniqueness of the pediatric population and describe how infants and children are similar or dissimilar to adults with regard to physiology, drug metabolism, immunology, cognitive effects, and response to disease states and therapy.

HISTORICAL BACKGROUND

Presented by Sumner Yaffe, M.D.
Director, Center for Research for Mothers and Children,
National Institute for Child Health and Human Development

Since passage of the Food and Drug Modernization Act of 1997 and subsequent revision of regulations by the U.S. Food and Drug Administration (FDA), children as a class of individuals have come a long way toward receiving better and more appropriately dosed therapeutics. One has to look back only to 1938 when sulfanilamide (called an elixir) appeared on the market as an antibacterial drug. Everyone was anxious to use it for infants and children, particularly for the treatment of infectious diseases prevalent among children at that time. The elixir, made by mixing sulfanilamide with diethylene glycol, was distributed for 1 month before 107 children died of renal toxicity following its administration.

In 1938 the Food and Drug and Cosmetic Act was amended to require premarketing clearance for new drug applications (NDAs). Drugs had to be safe but not necessarily efficacious. In 1960 the sedative thalidomide dramatically raised new issues about the importance of testing drug safety in a variety of populations and established the need to have standards for effectiveness. Additional requirements were enacted. Those requirements mandated that those submitting NDAs weigh the benefit versus the risk and conduct adequate and well-controlled clinical trials with full and informed consent. Despite the evolution of strict standards for the testing of drugs with adults, 80 percent of drugs that are on the market have not been tested in studies with children. Studies of drugs with infants and children are urgently needed. The agenda of this workshop emphasizes the unmet state of knowledge regarding drug action and disposition in the pediatric population. The need for further research is clearly identified. Modern molecular biology and genetics, when applied to pharmacologic studies in infants and children, will markedly advance our understanding of drug actions and enable us to practice rational therapeutics.

DIFFERENCES BETWEEN CHILDREN AND ADULTS

Presented by Ralph Kauffman, M.D.
*Director of Medical Research, Children's Mercy Hospital,
Kansas City, Missouri*

The rules by which practitioners have extrapolated adult drug doses to infants and children have not always been based on biologic or pharmacologic logic. Moreover, they have tended to be overly simplistic, in that they assume a linear relationship between children and adults and do not incorporate the complex, nonlinear changes in growth and development that take place during childhood.

Indeed, it is the dynamic process of growth, differentiation, and maturation that sets children apart from adults. In addition to growth in physical size, dramatic changes in body proportions, body composition, physiology, neurologic maturation, and psychosocial development take place during infancy and childhood. These changes are of equal if not greater importance than growth in physical size in terms of the child's development, response to disease, and response to therapeutic modalities.

Growth and development are particularly rapid during the first 2 years of life. Body weight typically doubles by 6 months of age and triples by the first birthday. Body length increases by 50 percent during the first year. Body surface area doubles during the first year. During this metamorphosis, major organ systems grow and mature. In the first 18 months of life the child becomes ambulatory, develops socialization skills, and learns verbal language. The other period of childhood when important changes take place is puberty, when accelerated growth and sexual maturation occur. In addition, body proportions continue to change significantly from childhood to adulthood.

The respective proportions of body weight contributed by fat, protein, and water change during infancy and childhood. At birth, total body water constitutes approximately 80 percent of body weight. By 5 months of age, however, total body water accounts for only 60 percent of body weight and then remains relatively constant. However, there is a progressive decrease in extracellular water throughout childhood and into young adulthood. As the proportion of body water decreases, the percentage of body weight contributed by fat doubles by 4 to 5 months of age. In addition, protein mass increases during the second year of life as the child becomes ambulatory.

Major organ systems change in relative size as well as function during childhood. For example, the weights of liver and kidneys—the major organs responsible for drug elimination—relative to body mass are several-fold greater in the preschool-age child than in young adults. Likewise, in preschool-age children, the ratio of body surface area to body weight, which reflects the relative size of the skin as an organ, is approximately 2.5 times that in adults.

A number of quantitative and qualitative differences in the anatomy and physiology of the infant and developing child can affect the absorption of various drugs and other xenobiotic compounds:

1. As with the skin area, the absorptive surface area of the gut is relatively greater in the infant than in the adult.
2. Gastric pH is 7 to 8 at birth and then falls to less than 3 during the first 1 to 2 hours of life. However, relative hypochlorhydria persists during the first 1 to 2 months of life. Premature infants have impaired gastric acid production until after 32 weeks of gestational age. This allows orally administered acid-labile drugs that may not be absorbed intact in the mature individual to have greater bioavailability in premature and very young infants.
3. The infant has decreased pancreatic exocrine function, which matures by the first year. This decreased function may affect the absorption of prodrug esters of fatty acids.
4. The immature gut also exhibits permeability to large molecular species, including intact proteins that are not absorbed by the mature gut.
5. Gastric emptying and gut transit time may be prolonged in premature and ill newborns. On the other hand, healthy infants may have transit times shorter than those for adults.
6. Infants have decreased first-pass metabolism of drugs, with increased levels of uptake until the metabolic pathways resident in the gut mucosa and liver mature. This may lead to greater bioavailability of drugs that undergo significant first-pass metabolism.

Protein binding of drugs can affect drug pharmacodynamics, toxicity, distribution, and elimination. Maturational differences in protein binding are primarily an issue during infancy:

1. Plasma protein binding of drugs typically is decreased in the newborn and young infant. This is most pronounced in the premature infant.
2. Decreased binding is attributed to decreased levels of circulating protein (albumin and α-1-glycoprotein) and also to a decreased affinity for certain ligands. In some cases, decreased binding may also be attributed to competition for binding sites with other drugs or highly bound endogenous substances. The ultimate effect on binding of a specific drug depends on the relative binding affinities and molar concentrations of the competing ligands.
3. Binding is also pH dependent and may be decreased in the presence of acidosis.
4. Developmental differences in drug binding may occur with tissue binding as well as with plasma proteins.*

---

*For example, in the mid-1970s, two groups demonstrated that digoxin binding to the myocardium was much greater in infants than in adults (Andersson et al., 1975;

Glomerular filtration (regulation of renal blood flow) rates and tubular transport mechanisms all are physiologically decreased at birth but increase rapidly during the first month of life and reach maturity before the end of the first year. Maturational changes in renal function have profound implications for administration of drugs that are primarily excreted by the kidney.

Puberty is another period in development that involves major physiologic changes, including (1) large growth spurts mediated by surges in human growth hormone and other growth factors, (2) increase in luteinizing hormone and follicle-stimulating hormone concentrations with secondary sexual maturation associated with the effects of estrogen or progesterone and testosterone, and (3) gender-specific changes in body composition, with females acquiring a greater proportion of body fat and males having larger lean muscle mass.

Children differ from adults not only in anatomic and physiologic ways but also in the types of diseases from which they suffer and in their manifestations of those diseases that they do have in common with adults. This can determine the types of therapies developed for children as well as the design of studies that test new therapeutic agents. In addition, some diseases occur only in children and therefore can only be studied by studies with children. For example, newborn respiratory distress syndrome is unique to the immature newborn. Clinical trials of surfactant for the prevention or treatment of the syndrome were conducted first and only with newborns, with no studies performed with subjects in other age groups. Other examples are bronchopulmonary dysplasia and retinopathy of prematurity, which are unique to premature infants. Consequently, new approaches to the amelioration of these conditions must necessarily be studied almost exclusively in studies with infants.

In addition, certain malignancies occur only in children, such as neuroblastoma and Wilms' tumor. Congenital heart defects are generally diagnosed and treated during infancy and childhood and exhibit a range of pathophysiologies and hemodynamics that are uncommon in adults.

Furthermore, certain infectious diseases, such as rubella, rubeola, mumps, pertussis, and *Haemophilus influenzae* infection occur primarily in childhood. Therefore, studies that document the efficacies of vaccines for the prevention of these infections must be carried out with healthy infants and young children. Data derived from studies with adults cannot be extrapolated to children. For example, in contrast to adults and older children, children under age 2 years did not develop protective immunity to *H. influenzae* from the first commercially available vaccine, because of differences in their immune responses. Subse-

---

Gorodischer et al., 1976). In addition to differences in myocardial binding, they showed a three fold greater erythrocyte binding of digoxin in infants than adults. These studies are highly suggestive of a developmental difference in the affinities of sodium and potassium-ATPases for digoxin.

quently, the conjugated vaccine, which confers immunity to children less than 12 months of age, was developed after appropriate evaluation in this age group.

In developing drugs for pediatric populations, investigators must recognize that some diseases that are superficially similar between children and adults may have very different pathophysiologies in children. For example, human immunodeficiency virus (HIV) infection and AIDS may occur at any age. However, it was realized within a few years after the start of the AIDS pandemic that the clinical course of the infection in infants differs in several important aspects from that in adults. It became apparent that the Centers for Disease Control and Prevention criteria for AIDS, developed out of experience with the adult population, did not apply to infants and young children. In addition, progression of the infection in infants tended to be more rapid than in adults. Before current antiviral therapies became available, survival times for children were shorter than those for adults. Studies focused on the pediatric age group led to advances in understanding of the pediatric manifestations of the disease, and these advances have led to major shifts in therapeutic approaches for infants and children with HIV infection.

As another example, hypertension occurs in infants and children as well as adults, although the dominant causes of hypertension are different between the two groups. Whereas most cases of hypertension in adults are classified as primary or essential, most cases of hypertension in children are secondary and are most commonly associated with renal disease. Essential hypertension is rarely identified until late childhood or adolescence. This has profound implications for the design of studies that test the effects of antihypertensive drugs in children and the choice of new antihypertensive drugs to be tested in studies with children.

Finally, children may be more or less vulnerable than adults to the adverse effects of drugs. This possibility must always be considered when designing a drug trial or developing a new drug for pediatric use. There have been numerous examples of greater or unpredictable vulnerability of children to adverse effects, including the following:

- An entire generation of children suffered enamel dysplasia from exposure to tetracycline antibiotics during critical periods of formation of dentition, an adverse effect that could never have been anticipated on the basis of data from clinical trials conducted with adult populations.
- Verapamil was given to infants to convert supraventricular tachycardia on the basis of experiences with adults. After a series of infant deaths associated with its use, the different response in infants was recognized and verapamil is no longer used for this indication in infants.
- Desflurane, an inhalation anesthetic, provides rapid, smooth, and safe anesthesia induction in adult patients and appeared to be an ideal anesthetic for children. However, in pediatric patients it causes an unacceptable incidence of laryngospasm, breath holding, and hypersecretion when used as an induction

agent. This life-threatening adverse event could not have been predicted from the results of trials with adults.

Conversely, children can be less vulnerable to adverse drug effects than adults. For example, infants are less susceptible to renal toxicity from aminoglycoside antibiotics, possibly due, in part, to a reduced ability to concentrate the drugs intracellularly in renal tubular and epithelial cells. In addition, hepatotoxicity from the general anesthetic halothane is relatively rare in children, whereas it is not uncommon in adults. As another example, the risk of isoniazid-induced hepatitis is negligible in children, whereas the reported incidence is 23 per 1,000 patients in middle-age adults.

Because children differ from adults in so many important aspects and are dependent on adults for their welfare, certain ethical and logistical issues must also be considered when designing and conducting research that involves children. The anatomic, physiologic, and psychologic dynamics of growth and development must be accommodated at various developmental stages. This frequently requires age-appropriate modification of approaches typically used in studies with adult subjects, particularly when obtaining informed consent and conducting risk-benefit analyses.

In terms of informed consent, children cannot independently consent to participate in research; thus, surrogate consent or permission must be provided by a parent or guardian. When gaining surrogate consent or authorization to participate in research, it is important to ensure that the child's interests are protected. It is essential to give the child with sufficient cognitive ability the opportunity to assent to participation.

When evaluating risks and potential benefits, investigators must consider the child's age, developmental status, and condition. For example, children at various ages have unique fears, anxieties, and perceptions of body threat that must be considered. To the young child, being in a strange environment and separated from parents may be a greater threat than the procedures directly related to the study. For the adolescent, perceived loss of privacy associated with, for example, urine collection may be a source of embarrassment that is far more threatening than venipuncture. It is therefore important to take whatever steps are feasible to minimize fear, anxiety, and discomfort associated with a study. In addition, consideration of parents' perceptions is important in terms of their views of the possible benefits versus risks and the amount of discomfort or inconvenience that they perceive their child will suffer by participation in the study.

Regarding the logistics of conducting studies with children, several issues deserve consideration. For example, if multiple blood samplings are required, there may be a need to use indwelling cannulae and to time research blood sampling so that it coincides with clinical sampling when possible. Acute blood loss should not exceed 3 percent of total blood volume, which can be quite limiting in younger children and infants. This may necessitate adapting assays to smaller clinical sample sizes. When developing outcome measures, assessment tools might have to be adapted so that they are applicable to younger age groups. For example, in conducting analgesic studies the same pain assessment methods used for a 25-year-old individual cannot be used for a 5-year-old child.

Finally, age-appropriate dose formulations must be considered. Palatable liquid formulations are preferable for orally administered medications for infants and young children. If solid dosage formulations must be administered, they may have to be administered with an age-appropriate food, and when doing so, the age of the child must be considered (e.g., infants cannot take the dosage with solid food).

In summary, growth and development add complexity to the already complex world of drug metabolism and pharmacodynamics. This process is neither simple nor linear. It should be obvious, then, that the results from studies with adults typically cannot be extrapolated to children. The younger the child, the more this is true. Studies of drugs for use in children must be designed to take into effect the complex developmental changes that can affect drug biodisposition and pharmacodynamics. Developmental effects may not always be predictable. As the gaps in knowledge are gradually and painstakingly filled in, the development of new therapeutic agents for children will be enhanced, drugs will be given to children with greater precision and safety, and in the end, infants and children will be the ultimate beneficiaries.

DIFFERENTIAL RESPONSES OF CHILDREN TO DRUGS

Presented by John T. Wilson, M.D.
Professor and Chief of Clinical Pharmacology, Department of Pediatrics, Louisiana State University Health Sciences Center, Shreveport

Past negative experiences with the differential responses of children to drugs—such as the deaths that occurred with elixir of sulfanilamide, tooth staining after tetracycline treatment, kernicterus after sulfisoxazole treatment, and cardiovascular collapse after chloramphenicol treatment—highlight the long-standing and sometimes severe effects that can occur when drugs are not properly studied before their use in children. Insufficient information about pediatric dosing prompted investigations of the pharmacokinetics and pharmacodynamics of drugs in children. This work with children and immature animals showed a maturational pattern for metabolic clearance of many drugs. The publication of the 1994 FDA Pediatric Rule and enactment of Section III of the Food and Drug Administration Modernization Act in 1997 allowed (1) extrapolations of information to children only when efficacy and drug action were similar in adults, and (2) a 6-month extension of patent exclusivity when a sponsor performed studies with children at the request of FDA. These actions exposed the need for the identification of differential drug responses in children and their underlying mechanisms and illustrated the need for clinical research in this area if extrapolations of information from studies with adults were to be made with validity. What was the extent and magnitude of a differential response, and how much harm had occurred from not knowing the proper pediatric dose? Answers to these and other questions proved difficult from a search with conventional literature index systems. To obtain this information in a structured format amenable to literature searches, the following classification system was developed and tested with existing data.

A hierarchical classification system has, for all its categories, a maturational base that can be inserted at any level to limit or expand the question being asked with regard to differential drug responses in children. The lower the insertion, the more focused the question. Some items in this base are absorption and disposition, pharmacodynamics, childhood diseases (action on or confounding by), and vulnerability of the affected locus (i.e., a window of maximum risk). The following are categories of the classification system:

1. Response. Drug response is divisible into efficacy (achieving the desired response to the drug) or safety; either or both components can be decreased, increased, or considered appropriate for children relative to adults. Safety issues tend to focus on side effects, idiosyncratic reactions, or toxicity in children.

2. Differentiation. An efficacy or safety response is differentiated in children by either intensity (quantitative) or type (qualitative). An intensity or type of reaction that is different in children compared with that in adults may occur and is customarily referenced against drug dose or concentration in plasma.

3. Characteristics. Additional sets of characteristics identify and describe differential drug responses in children: whether the response is overt or covert, immediate or delayed, acute or chronic, and temporary or permanent. A further description for each includes incidence, magnitude, confounding, and treatability.

4. Orientation. Lastly, responses are described with regard to orientation of the question to cause or outcome. Orientations include drug, clinical, or chemical event; outcome (or a surrogate marker for the desired clinical outcome); and direct or indirect cause. This classification system allows one to operationalize the relevant response differences as they relate to human maturation and the pharmacology of a drug. Applications of the classification system to known differential drug responses in children illustrate its utility.

Questions about differential efficacy are qualified according to intensity and confounded as they apply to antipyretics as a drug class. Febrile children show nonlinear pharmacodynamics (the initial temperature sets the extent of fall in temperature), a lag period between time of maximum level in plasma and response, and slope and cyclic functions embedded in the temperature response to pyrogen and drug (Brown et al., 1993, 1998; Wilson et al., 1982). This has not been shown for adults.

Another drug class to which efficacy, intensity, and magnitude have been applied is the antihypertensive class of drugs (angiotensin-coverting enzyme inhibitors and nifedipine). The efficacy, intensity, and acute action of a drug applied to a disease can be shown with theophylline. The effect of the drug diminishes with increasing severity of asthma. In addition, a delayed efficacy response is seen when hypothyroid children of different ages are given thyroid replacement. In contrast to delayed effects, however, a chronic characteristic is noted for many psychotropic drugs given to children with behavioral disorders.

When safety is the major consideration, categories 2 to 4 mentioned above assist in focusing on the question. That of high intensity, incidence, and of a delayed nature is illustrated by a skin rash that followed 5 to 7 days after children received a loading dose of phenytoin. It was found in approximately 54 percent of children and 5 to 10 percent of adults. A threshold in plasma was found and metabolite analysis allowed postulation of in situ (skin) metabolism that led to a rash in those children poor for formation of *p-hydroxyphenytoin* (Wilson et al., 1976, 1978). Anticonvulsant drug safety with regard to categories of type, overt actions, and drug class is shown by a paradoxical reaction to phenobarbital, an increase in absence seizures with carbamazepine, and worsening of cognition in children treated with valproic acid. A change on category 3 to temporary classifies pediatric safety concerns for benzodiazepines. Paradoxical reactions to diazepam, aggression with clonazepam, and disinhibition with midazolam are examples.

In sum, efficacy and safety components of study design should be strengthened by a structured classification system that yields data for analysis of differential drug responses in children. Although fundamental pharmacology studies with immature-animal models are useful, when it comes to determining qualitative or even quantitative differences in drug responses in children, it is essential that children be studied and that data be categorized in a way that facilitates their access in multiple ways when one asks questions about differential drug responses in children. It is hoped that indexing systems will incorporate this new classification so that much needed pediatric drug data can be filed, retrieved, and collated in a comprehensive manner.

MOLECULAR BASIS OF DRUG METABOLISM

Presented by Thierry Cresteil, Ph.D.
Institut Gustave Roussy, Villejuif, France

The ontogeny of drug-metabolizing enzymes in humans could explain several differences in the consequences of drug exposure in adult and pediatric populations. Obstetricians must be mindful of the teratogenic potential of drugs, pollutants, or toxic compounds, and pediatricians need to be attentive to the effects of maturation in modifying the pharmacokinetics and clearance of a drug or in impairing the elimination of endogenous molecules from the body.

North American and European studies have demonstrated that the average number of drugs ingested during pregnancy is 10.3, with the range being from 3 to 29. As a consequence, most infants have drugs and metabolites stored in their tissues in the microgram or milligram range after labor and parturition. A survey conducted in an intensive care unit revealed exposure to an average of 3.4 drugs per infant in neonatal practice, and exposure was generally inversely related to birth weight. Further exposure can occur through breast-feeding.

The knowledge of the biotransformation pathways that a drug undergoes in the human liver and the capacity of the fetal and neonatal liver to catalyze these reactions will allow one to predict the metabolic fate and the potential risk of drug toxicity at every stage of development.

Drug-Metabolizing System

In the human liver, a multienzyme system is responsible for the biotransformation of hydrophobic molecules. In a first step, hydrophobic molecules are converted by phase I enzymes and are further conjugated to cellular acceptors by phase II enzymes. The balance between phase I and II enzymes controls the accumulation of activated molecules in the cell and thus the formation of adducts to protein or DNA. Because of the wide variety of substrates, phase I and phase II enzymes exist as isoforms, with a partial and overlapping substrate specificity, which could be investigated in vitro with human liver microsomes.

Cytochromes P450 (P450 or CYP) are the major phase I enzymes and are mostly expressed in the liver but are expressed to a lesser extent in the intestine, kidneys, and lungs. In the adult human liver, more than 15 isoforms of P450 are expressed, but there is wide variability for a given isoform. These variations result from different genetic backgrounds and from heterogeneous chemical exposures among individuals. Some substrates are specific to a single isoform: for example, debrisoquine is hydroxylated only by CYP2D6. A majority of compounds, however, could undergo metabolism by several routes, each catalyzed by different enzymes, leading to the formation of metabolites with variable therapeutic or toxic capacities.

Lastly, the expression of these enzymes could be modulated by the administration of molecules capable of stimulating their synthesis. In addition to drugs like barbiturates or steroids, molecules present in the diet (e.g., alcohol or flavonoids) or in the environment (e.g., polycyclic aromatic hydrocarbons) could act as inducers of P450.

Ontogeny of Monooxygenase System

Yaffe and colleagues first described the monooxygenase activities in the human fetal liver in 1970. A few years later extensive studies by Pelkonen and coworkers (1973) demonstrated that the human fetal liver contained an appreciable amount of P450 and its associated electron transfer chain components and was able to actively carry out a variety of reactions. However, certain activities remained extremely low and suggested that P450s could develop independently in the liver (Pelkonen et al., 1973). By preparing antibodies against human P450s, it was determined by immunoblotting that CYP2C was absent from the fetal liver, whereas CYP3A was actively synthesized, a finding that emphasized the role of CYP3A during the fetal period (Cresteil et al., 1985).

Microsomes prepared from the fetal liver were active not only against exogenous drugs but also against endogenous compounds like lipids and a wide variety of steroids. In 1982 it was demonstrated that if the level of 6β-hydroxylation of testosterone was lower in the fetal liver than in the adult liver, the 16α-hydroxylation of dehydroepiandrosterone (DHEA) was several times higher in fetal liver preparations (Cresteil et al., 1982). Therefore, it was concluded that the major function of P450 in the fetal liver is to eliminate endogenous hydrophobic molecules. To confirm this information based on protein determinations, reverse transcription-polymerase chain reaction (RT-PCR) has been used to detect the presence of ribonucleic acids (RNAs) encoding P450 isoforms. In fetuses of 11 to 24 weeks of gestational age, no RNA coding for CYP1A, CYP2A, CYP2B, or CYP2E has been detected, whereas RNA encoding CYP3A was the major isoform found in the liver (Hakkola et al., 1994).

Exploration of Neonatal Period

To understand the ontogeny of P450 isoforms, the liver content of individual P450 proteins and RNA and the capacities of these proteins to metabolize endobiotic and xenobiotic compounds were investigated by using postmortem liver samples from newborns and children between the ages of 1 hour and 10 years who had died from various pathologies, such as infection, hypotrophy, malformation, respiratory distress, or sudden death. To eliminate the possible interaction of pathologies with the regulation of drug-metabolizing enzymes, the level of expression was carefully examined. In most cases the cause of death did not play a crucial role in the regulation of expression of the monooxygenase system. Similarly, infants receiving drugs known for their inductive capacity were excluded from the study. The total P450 content was shown to remain stable from the first trimester of gestation to 1 year of age and account for about 30 percent of the adult level (Treluyer et al., 1997).

CYP2C proteins were confirmed to be definitively absent from the fetal liver but to rise during the first week after birth, regardless of gestational age at birth. After 1 week the level of CYP2C remains fairly stable up to age 1 year but does not exceed 30 percent of the adult level.

Two enzymatic activities that depend on CYP2C—the hydroxylation of tolbutamide, and the demethylation of diazepam—were measured in these samples and were found to parallel the evolution and rise in the level of the protein content after birth. The coordinated increases in these enzymatic activities suggest that the two proteins are coregulated. This is also evidenced indirectly by the examination of the RNA contents of developing livers. RNAs coding for CYP2C8, CYP2C9, and CYP2C18 were individually estimated by RT-PCR: RNA for CYP2C9 was the predominant RNA synthesized in the liver but the levels of RNAs for CYP2C isoforms increased during the first week following birth. It is likely that the activation of CYP2C genes occurs during the first week after birth, promoting the synthesis of CYP2C proteins and related activities.

This early rise in the levels of CYP proteins in the liver was also confirmed with in vivo data. Urine samples from infants given diazepam for sedative purposes were collected and analyzed. The production of metabolites was very low in infants aged 1 to 2 days, was notably higher after 1 week of age, and then remained stable up to age 5 years (Treluyer et al., 1997).

The major P450 subfamily expressed in the human liver is the CYP3A subfamily, which comprises three isoforms: CYP3A4, CYP3A5, and CYP3A7. Although highly homologous in terms of protein sequence (CYP3A5 is 87 percent homologous to CYP3A7 and 84 percent homologous to CYP3A4), these proteins display different substrate specificities and different patterns of expression. Thus, CYP3A7 is mostly expressed in the fetal liver, whereas CYP3A4 is the major P450 isoform present in the adult liver, accounting for 40 percent of the total P450 content (Cresteil et al., 1985). In subsequent studies, CYP3A4, CYP3A5, and CYP3A7 were recognized by antiserum against CYP3A4: the amount of reacting material was similar in all samples, whatever the age of the child, indicating that the overall level of the three isoforms was nearly constant from the first third of gestation to adulthood (Lacroix et al., 1997).

To discriminate between CYP3A4 and CYP3A7 two approaches have been used

1. By using an oligonucleotide specific for CYP3A4, the amount of RNA was estimated. As expected, the CYP3A4 RNA content was low in fetuses and increased after birth to reach a plateau during the first week after birth.

2. Specific substrates were designed to probe the two proteins. For that purpose, CYP3A4, CYP3A5, and CYP3A7 have been cloned and transfected into a human-derived cell line. Expressed CYP3A7 is able to actively convert DHEA into its 16-hydroxy metabolite, whereas CYP3A4 retains a very low level of activity. The 6-hydroxylation of testosterone, which is extensively catalyzed by CYP3A4 and which is only moderately catalyzed by CYP3A7, is used to probe the CYP3A4 activity (Mäenpää et al., 1993). With these two sub-

strates the relative evolution of both proteins was estimated during the perinatal period. As expected, the activity of CYP3A4 was shown to rise during the first week after birth, whereas CYP3A7 exhibits a high level of activity in fetuses, is maximal during the first week after birth, and thereafter declines to reach an extremely low level in adults (Lacroix et al., 1997).

These studies confirm that recombinant P450 proteins retain the same catalytic properties as the native protein present in liver microsomes and suggest the suitability of this model for the prediction of biotransformation reactions. This model was further used to evaluate the hydroxylation of cortisol by liver microsomes, since this reaction of 6β-hydroxylation has been proposed as an index that can be used to probe CYP3A activity. Only the CYP3A4 protein and, to a lesser extent, the CYP3A5 protein are able to actively hydroxylate cortisol, whereas CYP3A7 exhibits a very low level of activity. This result contradicts a recent report in which the 6-hydroxy cortisol/cortisol ratio was high at birth and progressively declined at the moment when CYP3A4 is supposed to replace CYP3A7. To date there is no explanation for this discrepancy.

Another point to consider is the polymorphic expression of CYP3A5. Twenty to 25 percent of the adult population is positive for CYP3A5. The proportion of the fetal and neonatal populations who are positive is the same, indicating that the fraction of the population that expresses CYP3A5 is the same at all ages. As for CYP3A4, the surge in the CYP3A5 level occurs during the first week after birth, and the amount of protein detected in liver microsomes remains nearly constant during the first year of life.

For CYP1A2, the protein develops very late during the postnatal period: the first rise in the protein level is observed only during the 3 months after birth, progressively increasing into adulthood. The evolution of the protein is correlated with the increase in the associated enzymatic activities, such as the dealkylation of methoxy- and ethoxyresorufin (Sonnier and Cresteil, 1998).

This late evolution of the CYP1A2 protein was confirmed with several other substrates. For instance, caffeine could be demethylated by CYP1A2 and hydroxylated by 3A: when caffeine was incubated in vitro with liver microsomes, the C8 hydroxylation was active in fetal preparations, whereas the demethylation by CYP1A2 remained negligible before a rise in its level during the first trimester (Cazenave et al., 1994).

Other CYP proteins are expressed during the perinatal period. Thus, CYP4A which supports the hydroxylation of fatty acids, is present in the fetal liver and its levels increase immediately after birth to its final levels during the first days after birth, probably in relation to the hydrolysis of triglycerides and the release of fatty acids that occur during this period (Treluyer et al., 1996). This release of fatty acids could also play a role in the regulation of CYP2E1. The protein is absent from fetal samples and surges during the first hours following birth. It is well known that ketone bodies generated during fatty acid degradation act by stabilizing the CYP2E1 protein. It is likely that the high level of plasma ketone bodies during the first days after birth (which, in fact, correspond to those after a 3- to 4-day fasting for adults) is responsible for the sudden surge in CYP2E1 in the livers of newborns (Vieira et al., 1996, 1998). Finally, CYP2D6 and CYP2A6 levels rise during the first days or week following birth (Jacqz-Aigrain et al., 1993; Treluyer et al., 1991).

These data allow the classification of P450 isoforms into three groups according to their patterns of expression:

- the fetal group that includes CYP3A7 and CYP4A, which act on endogenous substrates (steroids and fatty acids) and which are implicated in the elimination of those substances from the body;
- an early neonatal group composed of a majority of P450s that develop quickly during the hours or days after birth; and
- the late neonatal protein CYP1A2.

Conclusions

The data presented here emphasize the role of phase I enzymes during the early neonatal period in the human liver and raise questions about the susceptibility of children to hazards in the food chain, drug intake, or chemical exposure. Enzymes expressed in the human liver early in life could activate or inactivate chemicals. Moreover, the relative intensities of the different pathways that drugs undergo could vary in relation to age. For example, the metabolism of imipramine leads to the formation of several derivatives: in adults, the major metabolite formed is desmethylimipramine, which is essentially formed by CYP1A2, whereas the hydroxylation at position 2 is supported by CYP2D6.

According to age, the metabolism of imipramine demonstrates the relative evolution of P450: in fetuses there is no CYP2D6 and no CYP1A2. The biotransformation of imipramine remains very low (Cresteil, 1999). Immediately after birth the levels of CYP2D6 increase and the level of formation of 2-hydroxy imipramine is significantly increased. Later, levels of CYP1A2 surge and the formation of the desmethyl derivative predominates. This demonstrates that the evolution of the different pathways that drugs undergo is related to the evolution of the P450 responsible for the reaction, which could differ between children and adults. This makes it hazardous to extrapolate data for adults to children. To conclude, the xenobiotic metabolizing system is well developed in the livers of human newborns and neonates. The levels of most phase I and II enzymes rise during the first weeks after birth, regardless of gestational age at birth. The capacity of the human liver to eliminate xenobiotic compounds during the neonatal period is effective and the intensity of biotransformation depends primarily on the level of maturation of phase I enzymes.

To anticipate the metabolic fate of chemicals in the developing liver, it is possible to use proteins expressed in eukaryotic cell expression system. This has been done with steroids as a model and could be extended to other drugs. For example, an antiprotease molecule is extensively metabolized in vitro by adult human liver microsomes into four derivatives. As shown with recombinant human P450 the metabolism seems to be mostly dependent on CYP3A4 and, to a lesser extent, on CYP2C9 and CYP3A5, whereas CYP3A7 has no or little activity. This could result in a low level of biotransformation in the fetal and early neonatal liver. A consequence could be that in the case of a pregnant woman treated with antiprotease, biotransformation in the fetal liver should be very limited.

With knowledge of the biotransformation pathway of a drug and the ontogenic profiles of CYP proteins, it becomes possible to predict the metabolism and to potentially estimate the risk of drug exposure during the perinatal period. However, these biochemical data can give only an estimation and require experimental confirmation before definitive conclusions can be reached about the therapeutic or toxicological effects of chemicals in developing beings.

GENE EXPRESSION AND ONTOGENY OF DRUG METABOLISM

J. Steven Leeder, Pharm.D., Ph.D.
Associate Professor of Pediatrics and Pharmacology,
Children's Mercy Hospital and Clinics

At present, there is significant interest in understanding how pharmacogenetics and pharmacogenomics may improve the knowledge of interindividual variability in the clinical responses to therapeutic agents. In the context of pediatric pharmacotherapy, genetic and environmental determinants of variability are superimposed on a changing background of developmental and maturational processes that add further complexity to the optimal use of medications. For example, the weight of a newborn will double by 5 months of age and triple by 1 year of age, whereas caloric expenditures increase three- to fourfold over this same period of time. Thus, it is not unlikely that other functions, such as drug biotransformation, will undergo profound changes in this period of rapid growth and development. Current knowledge related to the expression of drug-metabolizing enzymes in infants and children during the first year of life is reviewed below with a focus on the cytochromes P_{450} (CYPs).

For many years, it was considered dogma that drug biotransformation capability was limited at best in the fetus and newborn but increased over the first year of life to levels in toddlers and young children that generally exceeded the adult capacity. In fact, in several situations examination of clinical pharmacokinetic data has revealed discernible patterns of drug clearance that can be attributed to developmental differences in drug biotransformation. As knowledge of mammalian drug biotransformation processes has increased over the past few years, it has become apparent not only that there are developmental differences in expression among drug-metabolizing enzyme families (CYPs, glucuronosyltransferases, etc.) but that individual drug-metabolizing enzymes may have unique developmental profiles (Cresteil, 1998) that influence the therapeutic response, desired or undesired, to a given agent. Specific examples are discussed below.

The CYP3A subfamily consists of three members in humans: CYP3A4, CYP3A5, and CYP3A7. The term CYP3A refers to these isoforms in a collective sense since, historically, it has been difficult to differentiate one from the others on the basis of immunochemical or catalytic properties. Nevertheless, the human CYP3A subfamily is one of the most important drug-metabolizing families in humans. CYP3A4 is the major isoform expressed in adult liver (Schuetz et al., 1994) and intestine (Kolars et al., 1994) and is known to metabolize more than 50 different drugs of diverse chemical structure. CYP3A7 is predominantly expressed in fetal liver (Komori et al., 1990), whereas CYP3A5 is the major CYP3A isoform expressed in human kidney (Schuetz et al., 1992); in contrast, CYP3A5 is expressed in only 25 percent of liver samples (Schuetz et al., 1994). In vitro studies indicate that CYP3A7-dependent DHEA 16α-hydroxylase activity is very high in fetal liver and shows maximal activity in the early neonatal period with a progressive decline thereafter. In contrast, CYP3A4 activity as measured by testosterone 6β-hydroxylation is essentially absent from the fetal liver but increases during the first week of postnatal life (Lacroix et al., 1997).

Acquisition of CYP3A activity in vivo is largely inferred from studies of cortisol 6β-hydroxylation in newborns. Nakamura and colleagues (1998a) observed that the ratio of 6β-hydroxycortisol to free cortisol in spot urine samples obtained within 24 hours of birth was higher in term newborns (16.6 ± 1.9; $n = 39$) than in premature newborns (5.3 ± 0.9, $n = 42$; $p < .001$). Significant positive correlations were observed between the 6β-hydroxycortisol-to-free cortisol ratio and gestational age as well as, to a lesser extent, between the ratio and birth weight, suggesting that the level of CYP3A activity is higher in more mature infants. However, the ratio in term infants declined over the first 3 to 5 days after birth to levels comparable to those in premature infants and to levels similar to those observed in adults (Nakamura et al., 1998a). Subsequent work has revealed that the ratio of 6β-hydroxycortisol to free cortisol in the urine of mature infants on the day of birth is independent of that in the urine of their mothers and, presumably, therefore, is independent of maternal CYP3A activity (Nakamura et al., 1999). Although it appears that CYP3A4, CYP3A5, and CYP3A7 are all capable of hydroxylating cortisol in the 6β position, CYP3A4 appears to be 5.7- and 11.4-fold more active than CYP3A5 and CYP3A7, respectively (T. Cresteil, Institute Gustave Roussy, Villejuif, France, personal communication, May 28, 1999).

A literal interpretation of the in vivo data presented by Nakamura and colleagues (1998a, 1999) therefore implies that CYP3A4 activity is compromised in premature newborns, whereas in term newborns, CYP3A4 activity is highest on the day of birth, with a gradual decline during the postnatal period. The data for term newborns are in marked contrast to the in vitro data obtained with human fetal hepatic microsomes cited above (Lacroix et al., 1997). In this regard, concern has been raised that the urinary 6β-hydroxycortisol-to-free cortisol ratio in not an adequate representation of hepatic CYP3A activity (Watkins, 1994), and thus, developmental changes in renal CYP3A5 activity could conceivably account for the observed maturational profile of cortisol 6β-hydroxylation, a possibility that has not been addressed directly either in vitro or in vivo. On the other hand, pharmacokinetic studies of other drugs that can serve as markers of CYP3A activity, such as midazolam, indicate that CYP3A activity in newborns is indeed reduced compared with that in older infants.

When administered intravenously, midazolam clearance reflects the CYP3A activity in the liver (Kinirons et al., 1999). On the basis of data from a population study of intravenous midazolam pharmacokinetics in critically ill neonates (Burtin et al., 1994), it is apparent that although considerable interindividual variability in midazolam clearance exists in this patient population, clearance (and thus hepatic CYP3A activity) is markedly lower in neonates less than 39 weeks of gestation (1.2 ml/kg/min) and greater than 39 weeks of gestation (1.8 ml/kg/min) relative to the clearance of 9.1 ± 3.3 ml/kg/min observed in infants greater than 3 months of age (Payne et al., 1989). The finding of low concentrations of 1′-hydroxymidazolam in neonates (Burtin et al., 1994) provides further confirmation that functional CYP3A activity is limited in the newborn period.

The midazolam data cited above suggest that CYP3A activity increases approximately five fold over the first 3 months of life (Payne et al., 1989). Carbamazepine (CBZ) represents an additional therapeutic entity that can be used to follow the maturation of CYP3A function in children since the formation of its major metabolite, carbamazepine 10,11-epoxide (CBZ-E), is largely a CYP3A4-mediated process (Kerr et al., 1994). Data from therapeutic drug monitoring databases and pharmacokinetic studies indicate that the rate of CBZ clearance is greater in children than in adults (Pynnönen et al., 1977; Riva et al., 1985) necessitating the administration of higher doses (on a milligram-per-kilogram basis) to children to achieve and maintain therapeutic concentrations. Korinthenberg and colleagues (1994) demonstrated that the ratio of CBZ-E to CBZ in plasma decreases over a period of time spanning the first year of life to 15 years of age. Although factors other than CYP3A4 activity (i.e., microsomal epoxide hydrolase activity) may also influence this ratio, these data are consistent with increased CYP3A4 activity in early childhood, with a gradual decline to levels approximating those in adults occurring around adolescence.

Phenytoin is widely used for the treatment of seizure disorders in children and adults. Biotransformation of phenytoin to (S)-5-(4-hydroxyphenyl)-5-

phenylhydantoin (S-HPPH) by CYP2C9 and subsequent conjugation with glucuronic acid represent the principal metabolic pathway by which the drug is eliminated from the body. Phenytoin can also be metabolized by CYP2C19 to yield R-HPPH. Under normal conditions, 95 percent of the HPPH recovered in the urine is the CYP2C9 product S-HPPH (Fritz et al., 1987). However, as plasma phenytoin concentrations increase from 5 to 60 µM, the contribution of CYP2C19 to overall phenytoin biotransformation is estimated to increase three-fold (Bajpai et al., 1996). Nevertheless, changes in phenytoin pharmacokinetics during development provide some insight into the maturation of CYP2C9 function.

In preterm infants, the phenytoin half-life is prolonged and highly variable (75.4 ± 64.5 hours) relative to that in term infants less than 1 week postnatal age (20.7 ± 11.6 hours) or to that in term infants greater than 2 weeks of age (7.6 ± 3.5 hours) (Loughnan et al., 1977). In vitro, CYP2C9-mediated phenytoin metabolism is saturable (Bajpai et al., 1996). Bourgeois and Dodson observed that saturable phenytoin metabolism was not apparent until approximately 10 days postnatal age suggesting that the acquisition of functional CYP2C9 activity was delayed over this time period. Data derived from phenytoin dosage individualization procedures in Japanese children ages 6 months to 15 years indicate that the Michaelis-Menten parameter K_m, is less than 20 µM (5 µg/ml) in the majority of patients (Chiba et al., 1980). These data indicate that CYP2C9 is primarily responsible for phenytoin elimination in this population given that phenytoin K_m values determined in vitro are 5 and 70 µM for CYP2C9 and CYP2C19, respectively (Bajpai et al., 1996). The Japanese data further indicate that V_{max} values clearly decline as one approaches adolescence. Although changes in phenytoin bioavailability may also contribute to the latter finding, the investigators cite data indicating that the fractional excretion of HPPH in urine does not vary over the age range studied, thus implying that the observed decrease in V_{max} is a function of decreased CYP2C9 activity during childhood (Chiba et al., 1980). This fact would then account for the higher phenytoin dosage requirements (on the basis of body weight) in younger children compared with those in adults (Leff et al., 1986).

Caffeine and theophylline are two compounds that are widely used in infants and children. For both compounds, CYP1A2 is the primary route of metabolic clearance. For theophylline, clearance is considerably lower in infants at the time of birth but increases over time. Furthermore, immature infants have a very limited capacity to metabolize the drug, and the majority is excreted unchanged in the urine. CYP1A2-mediated metabolism to 1,3-dimethyluric acid becomes quantitatively more important with increasing age, a process that appears to be completed at about 5 to 6 months of age (Kraus et al., 1993). These changes in theophylline biotransformation are accompanied by increased dosage requirements over the first year of life (Nassif et al., 1981). Elimination of caffeine is also dependent upon CYP1A2 activity, and its developmental profile is similar to that of theophylline (Aranda et al., 1979; Le Guennec and Billon, 1987). Consistent with in vitro data (Cresteil, 1998), functional CYP1A2 activity is among the last of the P450 activities to be acquired by the newborn and appears to be further delayed in breast-fed infants (Le Guennec and Billon, 1987).

The ontogeny of CYP2D6 activity has not been well characterized to this point in time. Investigators have initiated a study designed to test the hypothesis that within the first year of life acquisition of CYP2D6 activity consistent with genotype is dependent upon both gestational age and postconceptional age. Dextromethorphan phenotyping (administration of 0.3 mg of dextromethorphan DM as Robitussin® Pediatric per kg of body weight after the last evening feed techniques) is conducted with infants during the first year of life at six points timed to coincide with well-baby visits to a primary care physician. Overnight urine recovered from diapers is analyzed by high-pressure liquid chromatography for levels of dextromethorphan and three metabolites. Although the data are preliminary and have not yet been subjected to peer review, data to date for 45 samples obtained 13.9 ± 2.9 (mean ± standard deviations) days after birth indicate that at this postnatal age, the CYP2D6 phenotype (ratio of dextromethorphan to dextrorphan in urine) is consistent with the corresponding genotype determined as described above. However, changes in the pattern of dextromethorphan metabolite excretion in urine suggest that maturation of CYP3A (possibly intestinal CYP3A) is delayed relative to that of hepatic CYP2D6, occurring over the first 4 months of life.

In summary, available information concerning the developmental regulation of individual CYP isoforms is inferred from pharmacokinetic studies of drugs considered to be model substrates for those particular CYP isoforms. In most cases, the data consist of serial measurements of the parent compound from which clearance is estimated and compared with values obtained for adults. Concurrent data for metabolites would be extremely valuable since the ability to characterize individual drug biotransformation pathways becomes more likely. Longitudinal phenotyping studies with healthy children and specific disease populations may help bridge the gap between preclinical in vitro drug biotransformation studies. Subsequent pharmacokinetic studies. These studies may provide important information concerning the effects of disease processes on drug disposition. Ultimately, the goal of developmental pharmacogenetic studies is to better understand the determinants of interindividual variability during childhood such that pharmacotherapeutics can truly be optimized for children of all ages.

3
Pharmacokinetics and Pharmacodynamics in Children versus Adults

Pharmacokinetics and pharmacodynamics are very different in children and adults. For the majority of drugs, in children as well as adults, a relationship exists between pharmacokinetics and pharmacodynamics. The pharmacokinetics of many drugs vary with age (Kearns, 1998). For instance, because of the rapid changes in size, body composition, and organ function that occur during the first year of life, clinicians as well as pharmacokineticists and toxicologists are presented with challenges in prescribing safe and effective doses of therapeutic agents (Milsap and Jusko, 1994). Studies with adolescents reveal even more complexity in drug metabolism and differences in drug metabolism between the sexes.

The therapeutic value of understanding differences in pharmacokinetics because of developmental factors thus relies on an ability to understand better the dose versus concentration versus effect profile for a specific drug in patients of various ages (Kearns, 1998). In turn, recognition of differences in pharmacokinetics because of developmental factors can be invaluable for interpretation of data and improving and guiding the design of clinical trials on drug disposition and efficacy. The summaries of the presentations presented below identify new advances in biomedical science that are uniquely applicable to children and that could be applied to the development and testing of drugs and biologics in studies with children. Some of the challenges and successes in pediatric pharmacokinetics for particular studies are also discussed.

DRUG METABOLISM IN CHILDREN AND ADOLESCENTS: INSIGHTS FROM THERAPEUTIC ADVENTURES

Presented by Gregory L. Kearns, Pharm.D., FCP
Marion Merrell Dow/Missouri Chair in Pediatric Pharmacology, and Professor of Pediatrics and Pharmacology, University of Missouri, Kansas City, and Chief, Division of Pediatric Clinical Pharmacology and Experimental Therapeutics, Children's Mercy Hospital and Clinics, Kansas City

Over the past two decades, much information concerning drug metabolism in infants, children, and adolescents has been derived as a "by-product" of pharmacokinetic investigations designed, in part, to determine whether age-dependent differences in drug disposition (e.g., drug clearance) were evident. For many compounds, developmental differences in drug clearance have, for drugs where the primary biotransformation pathways are known, produced partial developmental "road maps" that have provided information on the patterns of ontogeny for important drug-metabolizing enzymes.

The use of pharmacokinetic data to examine the ontogeny of a drug-metabolizing enzyme is well illustrated by theophylline, a pharmacologic substrate for the P450 cytochrome CYP1A2. In 1981, Nassif et al. reported that the elimination half-lives of theophylline ranged between 9 and 18 hours in term infants 6 to 12 weeks of postnatal age. Furthermore, those investigators found a linear relationship between postnatal age and theophylline half-life, with values declining to approximately 3 to 4 hours by 48 weeks of life. Over a decade later, Kraus et al. (1993) demonstrated that the dramatic alterations in theophylline plasma clearance occurring between 30 weeks (i.e., approximately 10 ml/h/kg) and 100 weeks (i.e., approximagely 80 ml/h/kg) of postconceptional age was primarily the result of age-dependent differences in the metabolism of theophylline by CYP1A2 were dependent pathways. Further characterization of theophylline biotransformation in humans by Tjia et al. (1996) demonstrated that theophylline was adequate for use as a pharmacologic "probe" for the assessment of CYP1A2 activity given that approximately 80 percent of the formation of 1,3–dimethyluric acid at theophylline concentrations of 100 micromolar (μM) was catalyzed by this P450 isoform. Recently, Tateishi et al. (1999) administered theophylline to 51 pediatric patients ranging in age from 1 month to 14 years of age and examined the urinary ratios of three metabolites: 1-methyluric acid, 3-methylxanthine, and 1,3-dimethyluric acid. Examination of the urinary ratio of 1,3-dimethyluric acid to either 3-methylxanthine or 1-methyluric acid (both of which are generated by CYP1A2) demonstrated that CYP1A2 activity as competent as that of adults was reached by 3 months of postnatal age, a finding that corroborated earlier studies of the pharmacokinetics of the drug in infants (Kraus et al., 1993). Although these data collectively appear to have created a well-defined pattern of CYP1A2 ontogeny, early studies by Lambert et al. (1986) and a recent investigation by Gotschall et al. (1999a) demonstrated that both puberty and cystic fibrosis, respectively, influence the pattern of CYP1A2 ontogeny (reflected by the use of methylxanthines as probe compounds) and, thus, implicate sexual maturation and disease as potentially important co-variates for the expression of this particular cytochrome P450 during development.

Another example where pharmacokinetic data have shed important insights on the impact of development on drug metabolism resides with CYP3A4; the most abundant cytochrome P450 isoform in the human body which is responsible for catalyzing the biotransformation of well over 20 drugs commonly used in pediatric practice (Leeder and Kearns, 1997). As recently reviewed by de Wildt et al. (1999b), ontogeny appears to have a major impact on the activity of CYP3A4. Like the activity of CYP1A2, CYP3A4 activity appears to be greater in infants and children than in adults. A study of carbamazepine and carbamazepine 10,11-epoxide (a CYP3A4 product) conducted in infants and children 2 weeks to 15 years of age demonstrated an age-dependent decrease in the ratio of the epoxide metabolite to the parent drug in serum (Korinthenberg et al., 1994). These data suggest a higher level of CYP3A4 activity in children and a gradual maturation to adult levels of activity during adolescence; however, variability in the activity of microsomal epoxide hydrolase, which further catalyzes the biotransformation of the 10,11-epoxide to the corresponding *trans*-dihydrodiol may confound interpretation of the data (Kroetz et al., 1993). Additionally, increased CYP3A4 activity in young children is supported by clinical investigations of cyclosporine which have demonstrated pharmacokinetic differences of a magnitude sufficient to affect both dosing regimen and drug efficacy (Wandstrat et al., 1989). In contrast to other P450 cytochromes such as CYP1A2 and CYP2C9, neither gender nor menstrual cycle appears to alter the activity of CYP3A4, as assessed with either hepatic microsomal samples (Transon et al., 1996) or the in vivo pharmacologic probe midazolam (Kashuba et al., 1998).

With respect to the impact of ontogeny on CYP3A4 activity, the most dramatic differences appear to occur during the first 6 months of life. As recently demonstrated by Lacroix et al. (1997) in an in vitro study (oligonucleotide probes for detection of messenger ribonuclease acid [mRNA], immunoblot analysis for quantitation of CYP3A protein, and biotransformation of the CYP3A substrates dehydroepiandrosterone [DHEA] and midazolam) with human liver microsomes obtained from fetuses, neonates, infants, and children, CYP3A4 expression is transcriptionally activated during the first week of life and is accompanied by a simultaneous decrease in the level of CYP3A7 expression. Additionally, they demonstrated that CYP3A4 activity was extremely low in the fetus and attained 30 to 40 percent of adult activity at 1 month. This investigation demonstrated that adult levels of CYP3A4 were attained sometime between 3 and 12 months of postnatal age.

Pharmacokinetic evidence for this pattern of CYP3A4 ontogeny is reflected by studies with midazolam, a pharmacologic probe that enables assessment of both hepatic and intestinal CYP3A4/5 activity, depending upon the route of administration (i.e., intravenous route = hepatic activity; oral route = hepatic route and intestinal activity) (Thummel et al., 1996). As demonstrated by Burtin et al., (1994) (Figure 3-1), the uncorrected (i.e., in liters per hour) plasma clearance of midazolam at birth was directly correlated with birth weight, a surrogate measure for CYP3A4 competence. These data suggest that CYP3A4 activity increases approximately fivefold over the first 3 months of life and corroborate the in vitro findings of Lacroix et al. (1997). This pattern of the development of CYP3A4 activity postnatally can be expected to significantly alter the pharmacokinetics and potentially, the pharmacodynamics of cisapride, a prokinetic agent drug widely used in infants during the first year of life whose biotransformation is dependent upon CYP3A4 activity (Gotschall et al., 1999b). Finally, pharmacokinetic studies of the CYP3A4 substrates nifedipine, lidocaine, cyclosporine, and tacrolimus illustrate the profound and clinically important impact of ontogeny on CYP3A4 activity and potentially, for some drugs that are also substrates for p-glycoprotein, the impact of development on the activity of this drug transporter (de Wildt et al., 1999a).

In addition to CYP1A2 and CYP3A4, there is pharmacokinetic evidence that supports a developmental dependence in the activity of CYP2C9. Biotransformation of phenytoin to the (S)-5-(4-hydroxyphenyl)-5-phenylhydantoin (S-HPPH) by CYP2C9 and subsequent conjugation with glucuronic acid represents the principal metabolic pathway by which the drug is eliminated from the body. Under normal conditions, 95 percent of the HPPH recovered in the urine is the CYP2C9 product S-HPPH (Bajpai et al., 1996). However, as plasma phenytoin concentrations increase from 5 to 60 μM, the contribution of CYP2C19 to overall phenytoin biotransformation is estimated to increase threefold (Bajpai et al., 1996). Nevertheless, changes in phenytoin pharmacokinetics during development provide some insight into the maturation of CYP2C9. Specifically, phenytoin pharmacokinetic data reported by Chiba et al. (1980) three decades ago demonstrated an age dependence in V_{max}, which declined from approximately 14.0 mg/kg/day at 6 months of age to 8 mg/kg/day at 16 years of age. These changes were not associated with age-associated differences in the urinary excretion of HPPH. As well, recent pharmacokinetic data for the CYP2C9 substrate ibuprofen collected from 26 patients with cystic fibrosis ranging in age from 5.5 to 29.6 years demonstrated an inverse linear correlation between age and the apparent oral clearance of the drug (Kearns et al. 1999).

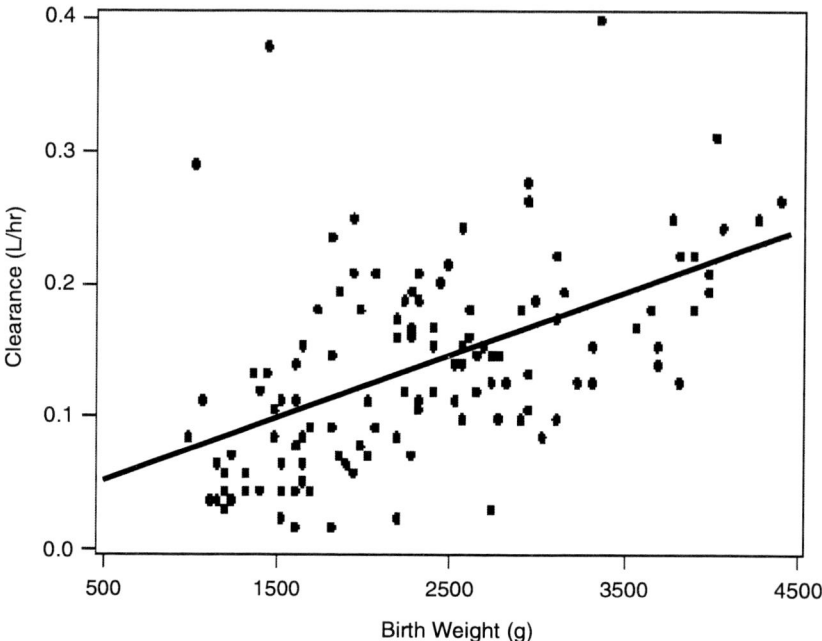

FIGURE 3-1 Midazolam clearance in newborns by birth weight. SOURCE: Reprinted, with permission, from Burtin et al. (1994, p. 620). © 1994 by Mosby–Year Book, Inc.

In addition to the P450 cytochromes, apparent age dependence exists for several phase II enzymes that are of quantitative importance for drug biotransformation (Leeder and Kearns, 1997). Studies of N-acetyltransferase 2 (NAT2) activity using caffeine as a pharmacologic probe demonstrated attainment of adult activity by approximately 4 to 6 months of postnatal age (Pariente-Khayat et al., 1991). In contrast, the activity of thiopurine methyltransferase (TPMT) in newborn infants is approximately 50 percent higher than that observed in adults (Pariente-Khayat et al., 1991), with no discernible correlation with age demonstrated for a group of 309 Korean children between 7 and 9 years of age (McLeod et al., 1995). Studies of the pharmacokinetics of drugs that are substrates for various sulfotransferase isoforms (e.g., acetaminophen) suggest that activity of this enzyme during infancy and early childhood exceeds levels in adults (Leeder and Kearns, 1997). Finally, as recently reviewed by de Wildt et al. (1999b), ontogeny appears to have a profound effect on the activities of several isoforms of uridine-5'-diphosphate (UDP)-glucuronosyltransferases (UGTs).

Studies that have examined the effect of age on the disposition of several UGT substrates (e.g., morphine, acetaminophen, ethinylestradiol, zidovudine, propofol, lorazepam, naloxone, diclofenac, bilirubin, and chloramphenicol) suggest that isoform-specific, age-related differences in UGT activity occur. For example, investigations of the pharmacokinetics of selected substrates for UGT2B7 (e.g., lorazepam, morphine and naloxone, chloramphenicol) support a marked reduction in the level of activity for this isoform (i.e., approximately 10 to 20 percent of the levels in adults) around birth, with attainment of competence equivalent to that in adults between 2 months and 3 years of age (de Wildt et al., 1999b). For drugs such as morphine, where UGT2B7 catalyzes the biotransformation of the drug to an active metabolite (e.g., morphine-6-glucuronide), delayed acquisition of morphine glucuronidation may have pharmacodynamic ramifications in the newborn as well. Available data concerning acetaminophen, a substrate for UGT1A6 and, to a lesser extent, UGT1A9, in children and adults suggest that the activities of these isoforms do not reach those in adults until 10 years of age (de Wildt et al., 1999b). Despite these examples, current data for the UGTs do not permit the construction of a developmental profile for these enzymes like those available for certain cytochromes P450 (e.g., CYP1A2, and CYP3A4). An information gap currently exists regarding the developmental and genetic aspects (i.e., the possible role of polymorphisms) of UGT regulation and its potential effect on pediatric drug therapy.

Despite a relative wealth of pharmacokinetic data and emerging information on isoform-specific differences in the activities of several important drug-metabolizing enzymes across the pediatric age range, there is little to no evidence that clearly describes the regulatory events at a cellular or molecular level that are responsible for producing developmental differences in drug metabolizing enzyme activity. Although it was commonly believed that age-dependent differences in hepatic size (relative to total body size) in children was in part responsible for the apparent increased activities of many drug-metabolizing enzymes during childhood, Murry et al. (1995) demonstrated that liver volume in 16 children (3.3 to 18.8 years of age) was not associated with changes in the normalized (i.e., normalized to weight or body surface area) clearance of lorazepam, antipyrine, or indocyanine green, from plasma. In a recent study, Relling et al. (1999) examined the catalytic activities of selected pharmacologic substrates (e.g., ethoxyresorufin for CYP1A2, ethoxycoumarin for CYP2E1, midazolam or teniposide for CYP3A4/5, tolbutamide for CYP2C9 and 17α-hydroxylation of paclitaxel for CYP2C8) using hepatic microsomes obtained from children ($n = 13$; 0.5 to 9.0 years of age) and adults ($n = 18$; 13 to 52 years of age). With the exception of the slightly lower CYP2C9 activity found for children than for adults, no significant age-related differences were noted for the remainder of the P450 cytochromes when catalytic activity was examined as a maximal rate per milligram of microsomal protein. Thus, apparent increases in the activities of selected P450 cytochrome reflected by pharmacokinetic studies of certain "substrates" do not appear to be supported by these in vitro findings.

Finally, it is possible that neuroendocrine determinants of growth and maturation may, in part, be responsible for the observed developmental differences in the activities of certain drug-metabolizing enzymes. As recently postulated by

Leeder and Kearns (1997), the biological effects of human growth hormone expressed during development may account for observed differences in the activity of specific drug metabolizing enzymes. Support for this assertion was drawn from evidence that human growth hormone can modulate the effect of many general transcription factors, the demonstrated regulatory role for growth hormone in the expression of CYP2A2 and CYP3A2 in rats, the documented effects of human growth hormone treatment on the alteration of the pharmacokinetics for pharmacologic substrates of selected P450 cytochromes, and also from evidence of altered CYP1A2 activity that appears to correlate with the pubertal height spurt (Lambert et al., 1986).

In conclusion, pharmacologic and pharmacokinetic evidence supports the presence of isoform-specific developmental differences in the activities of a host of phase I and phase II drug-metabolizing enzymes. In vitro characterization of pathways for human drug metabolism combined with in vivo confirmation of quantitatively important age-related differences in drug clearance can be used together to create an effective "pattern" to examine potential developmental "breakpoints" for drug metabolism. When this approach is effectively combined with a pharmacogenetic or pharmacogenomic assessment for enzymes that are polymorphically expressed, prediction of the impact of development on drug metabolism and disposition is possible. Such data can be used to guide pharmacokinetic simulations of clinical trials and are being effectively used to design Phase 1and 2 clinical trials of new drugs for infants, children, and adolescents. These experimental approaches will ultimately improve pediatric drug development by focusing the pharmacologically (and biologically) relevant questions for study, streamlining the design of clinical investigations (e.g., the study of targeted pediatric populations versus the entire pediatric population), and providing increasing opportunities to control drug exposure, a determinant of both drug efficacy and safety, through enhanced design of age (i.e., developmentally)-appropriate drug dosing regimens.

The translation of data concerning developmental differences in drug metabolism to the therapeutic arena poses interesting and, in some cases, formidable challenges. Specifically, it is important to recognize that many therapeutic drugs are polyfunctional substrates for drug-metabolizing enzymes. Hence, pharmacogenetic differences between patients of the same age can have profound effects on drug metabolism (and clearance) by producing quantitatively important differences in the rates and routes of drug biotransformation. Furthermore, the apparent drug biotransformation phenotype may be influenced by disease (e.g., infection), environmental factors (e.g., diet and environmental xenobiotics compounds), and concurrent medications. Also, it must be recognized that drug response is a function of the complex interplay among genes involved in drug transport, drug biotransformation, and receptor and signal transduction processes, among others.

Finally, it is imperative that future research in the area of developmental pharmacology be focused on defining at a whole-animal, molecular, and cellular level the regulatory events that produce the age-associated differences in the activities of drug-metabolizing enzymes. Clinical investigations designed to examine pharmacokinetics must include both genotypic and phenotypic assessments so that valid biologic correlates are available to address variability in both drug disposition and, in some cases, drug response. Translational and basic research must focus on the regulatory elements of those genes that control the expression of drug-metabolizing enzymes. Such a multifaceted approach will be necessary to characterize the dynamic changes in the activities of drug-metabolizing enzymes that characterize the period of human development.

ONTOGENY OF P-GLYCOPROTEIN, AN ATP-DEPENDENT TRANSMEMBRANE EFFLUX PUMP

Presented by Jon Watchko, M.D.
Associate Professor of Pediatrics, Obstetrics, Gynecology, and Reproductive Science, Department of Pediatrics, University of Pittsburgh School of Medicine

A common problem in newborns is neonatal unconjugated hyperbilirubinemia. Although generally a benign developmental phenomenon, hyperbilirubinemia can become severe, particularly in the context of underlying hemolytic disorders and prematurity. In survivors it can result in kernicterus (also called hyperbilirubinemic encephalopathy) and neurologic injury, which can produce profound, long-term neurodevelopmental sequelae. Central to the development of kernicterus is the passage of bilirubin across the blood-brain barrier into the central nervous system. It is believed that bilirubin can enter the brain when it is not bound to albumin (i.e., when it is free) by passive diffusion or when the blood-brain barrier is disrupted.

Despite its high affinity for membrane lipids, bilirubin demonstrates a low level of accumulation in the brain. In this respect, bilirubin is similar to other lipophilic compounds that share its characteristic of unexpectedly low levels of accumulation in the central nervous system.

Evidence suggests that bilirubin is an endogenously generated substrate for P-glycoprotein. The expression of P-glycoprotein in brain capillary endothelial cells may play a protective role in limiting the uptake of bilirubin into the central nervous system and thus plays a role in the pathogenesis of protecting against the genesis of kernicterus (hyperbilirubinemic encephalopathy).

P-glycoprotein is expressed constitutively in many tissues, including abundant expression in the luminal aspect of brain capillary endothelial cells in the blood-brain barrier and in the brush-border epithelial cells of the small intestine. With respect to the central nervous system, P-glycoprotein limits the influx and central nervous system retention of a wide variety of unrelated lipophilic compounds. Thus, P-glycoprotein contributes to the obstructive function of the blood-brain barrier by excluding compounds that are potentially toxic to the brain or extruding them before they have a chance to exert their cytotoxic effects. This includes the antiparasitic compound ivermectin, a well-defined P-glycoprotein substrate, various chemotherapeutic agents, and other potential neurotoxicants.

P-glycoprotein is a member of the adenosine triphosphate ATP-binding cassette or ABC superfamily of transport proteins that use ATP to translocate substrates across biologic membranes. It is encoded by a family of genes referred to as the multiple-drug resistance (MDR) genes because of their important role in contributing to resistance to multiple chemotherapeutic agents.

The MDR genes in humans are clustered on chromosome 7. The *mdr*1A gene encodes the P-glycoprotein isoform expressed in brain microvessels and confers a an MDR phenotype on tumors. This has two homologous halves, each of which has six hydrophobic transmembrane domains and an ATP-binding site. P-glycoprotein acts as an efflux pump, moving substrates across membranes against the concentration gradient. This has been demonstrated in tumor cells: approximately 60 percent of all tumors—solid or hematogenous—express P-glycoprotein. This has also been demonstrated in cell lines transfected with P-glycoprotein complementary deoxyribonucleic acids (cDNAs) and proteolysosomes reconstituted with P-glycoprotein.

The mechanism of action of P-glycoprotein primarily appears to be that of extracting substrates directly out of the plasma membranes before they get into the cell. Secondarily, P-glycoprotein can reduce intracellular substrate retention by pumping it out of the cell. The dependence of P-glycoprotein on ATP is absolute. P-glycoprotein has intrinsic ATP activity that can be distinguished from other ion motive ATPs and membrane-associated phosphatases. It is, in fact, stimulated by the addition of P-glycoprotein substrates. The ability of compounds to stimulate P-glycoprotein ATPase activity is directly correlated with their ability to be transported by the P-glycoprotein efflux pump. This pumping activity can be abolished by sodium azide, glucose deprivation, and mutations of the P-glycoprotein ATP-binding site.

One of the distinctive features of P-glycoprotein is its broad substrate specificity. Most of the substrates are lipophilic and amphipathic in nature, and virtually all are natural products of plants or microorganisms or are semisynthetic derivatives of such compounds. Known substrates for P-glycoprotein include the vinca alkaloids, anthracyclines, and other chemotherapeutic agents including taxol and cyclosporine; cardiovascular agents such as verapamil, digoxin, and quinidine; antibiotics; and various hormones.

Evidence suggests that bilirubin is a substrate for P-glycoprotein. This is based on observations that bilirubin will inhibit the photoaffinity labeling of P-glycoprotein by P-glycoprotein-specific photoaffinity probes. There is limited uptake of the tritiated bilirubin by human variant multiple-drug-resistant cells compared with that by parent cells that do not express the *mdr*1A gene. (See discussion below.) Watchko and colleagues are testing the hypothesis that the brain capillary endothelial cell P-glycoprotein may provide an important protective effect against bilirubin toxicity by reducing brain bilirubin influx.

Additional evidence that bilirubin is a P-glycoprotein substrate includes work on brain bilirubin content in wild-type versus transgenic *mdr*1A null mutant P-glycoprotein deficient mice (Watchko et al., 1998). The *mdr*1A null mutant mice do not express P-glycoprotein in brain capillary endothelium, whereas their *fvb* wild-type counterparts express P-glycoprotein in abundance, as determined by both immunohistochemical staining and the Western immunoblotting technique.

With the exception of the P-glycoprotein deficiency, the integrity of the blood-brain barrier is actually maintained in the *mdr*1A null mutant mouse line. There is no difference in blood-brain barrier permeability to non-P-glycoprotein substrates, including fluorocine and fluorocine dextran 4000 and other blood-brain barrier integrity markers. Rhodamine 123, which is a well-defined P-glycoprotein substrate, evinces a fourfold higher concentration of P-glycoprotein in the brain, *mdr*1A null mutant P-glycoprotein-deficient mice than in the brains of their *fvb* counterparts, without differences in blood levels.

Imaging studies demonstrate that only radio-labeled or technetium-labeled P-glycoprotein substrates show enhanced accumulation in the central nervous system in vivo in the null mutant. Thus, the P-glycoprotein that crosses the blood-brain barrier may provide a protective effect against bilirubin neurotoxicity by reducing bilirubin influxinto the brain.

To understand the potential effects within the neonatal period, when the risks for hyperbilirubinemic encephalopathy seem to be the greatest, the ontogeny of brain microvessel P-glycoprotein expression must be explored. Brain microvessel P-glycoprotein expression may in fact be an early marker of blood-brain barrier development. Studies with mice have demonstrated that P-glycoprotein expression in mouse brain microvessels is limited during late embryogenesis to the newborn period, and that brain microvessel expression increases markedly with postnatal maturation. Thus, low levels of P-glycoprotein expression in the immature brain may lead to enhanced bilirubin uptake by the brain and an increased risk for hyperbilirubinemic encephalopathy in newborns. P-glycoprotein expression in the intestine is also characterized by a marked increase with postnatal maturation.

The *mdr*1A gene modulates the developmental expression of P-glycoprotein. It is known that the *mdr*1A gene is differentially expressed in normal tissues in adults and is subject to modulation by factors such as the presence of heat shock. Glucocorticoids are known to increase *mdr*1A gene expression in the liver and lungs in the adult. Little is known about the effects of thyroid status on *mdr*1A gene expression.

Preliminary studies are addressing the perinatal factors that may modulate P-glycoprotein expression, specifically, the effects of uteroplacental insufficiency on P-glycoprotein expression. Models have shown that both the gene message and protein levels are decreased by about 50 percent in the case of uteroplacental insufficiency. Thus, an intrauterine milieu induced by uteroplacental insufficiency and characterized by hypoxia acidosis and altered metabolic fuel availability is associated with a significant reduction in brain microvessel P-glycoprotein expression. These findings are of interest in relation to understanding hyperbilirubinemic encephalopathy because alleged risk factors for kernicterus include hypoxia and acidosis, and the understanding that P-glycoprotein may limit the next influx of various lipophilic compounds, including bilirubin into the central nervous system.

Factors that will alter P-glycoprotein once it is expressed include chemosensitizers, multiple-drug-resistant antagonists, or MDR reversers. These compounds will compete for P-glycoprotein binding sites and inhibit P-glycoprotein activity, and thus will limit the effectiveness of P-glycoprotein as an efflux pump. Oncologists are interested in these compounds because by attenuating the MDR phenotype they can enhance the effectiveness of the various chemotherapeutic regimens.

In sum, these findings raise more questions than answers. The following questions warrant further investigation: (1) What are the functional consequences of these developmental variations in P-glycoprotein expression in normal tissues? (2) What role does intestinal P-glycoprotein play in determining drug oral bioavailability? (3) Is there individual variability in P-glycoprotein expression as a function of gender, ethnicity, or aging? (4) Are other related transporters, such as MDR-associated protein, MDR-associated protein type II, or the canalicular multiple organic transporter in the liver also subject to developmental modulation and do they affect drug absorption, metabolism, and disposition in the neonate?

DEVELOPMENTAL ASPECTS OF GLUCOSE TRANSPORTERS

Sherin U. Devaskar, M.D.
Vice Chair of Research, Department of Pediatrics, Division of Neonatology, Mattel Children's Hospital, University of California at Los Angeles

Glucose transport is a stereospecific, saturable, carrier-mediated process of diffusion. Studies to date have primarily measured glucose transport through various glucose analogues: 2-deoxyglucose uptake and 3-*O*-methylglucose transport. Recently studies with humans have used 18F-deoxyglucose uptake and positron emission tomography scanning to quantify glucose uptake in both the brain and skeletal muscle.

The carrier responsible for glucose transport is classified as either the sodium glucose cotransporter or the facilitative glucose transporter. The gene of a facilitative glucose transporter has about 10 to 11 exons, depending on the isoform. The protein, a 450-amino-acid peptide, is highly conserved between species and isoforms (five proteins that have been cloned and described to date). The glucose transporter Glut-1 is responsible for basal glucose transport. It has a KM (Michaelis constant) ranging from 1 to 5 milliMolar, is present in many tissues, represents a proliferative state, and is found in fetal tissues.

Glut-2, the isoform found in the liver, the beta cells of the pancreas, and the small gut has a higher KM of about 20 to 60mM. Glut-3, which is the third isoform, is found in the brain and the placenta and is thought to be the most efficient glucose transporter, with the lowest KM for glucose. Most of the studies that have been done thus far with adults have been with Glut-4, which is the insulin-responsive type of transporter, and is found only in insulin-responsive tissues, with a KM of about 5mM. Glut-5 is a fructose transporter. Glut-6, which was cloned and which was thought to be very closely related to Glut-3, turned out to be a pseudogene. The isoforms are substrate specific, and they are not alternatively spliced products. The genes for these proteins are separate and are located on different chromosomes. Their glucose kinetics match the requirements of the tissues in which they are expressed; thus, there is tissue-specific expression. In addition, they all demonstrate a developmental pattern of expression.

Studies with animals and human autopsy tissue have found that through development, Glut-1 is found in excess, particularly in the fetus, the newborn, and most tissues that have been examined, but levels decrease with advancing age. In contrast, with advancing age there is an increase in the levels of the liver (Glut-2), brain (Glut-3), and insulin-responsive (Glut-4) forms compared with the level of Glut-1.

Glut-4 serves as a useful marker of differences in insulin responsiveness that can occur over the lifetime of an individual. For example, very little Glut-4 is present in the fetal myocardium, compared with the amount present in the adult. In the fetal heart, Glut-1 is responsible for basal glucose transport. There is a dramatic decline in Glut-4 levels in the fetus of the severely diabetic mother. Similar findings were also obtained for the skeletal muscle of the fetus, which behaved exactly like the heart with respect to Glut-1 and Glut-4. Sheep models demonstrate that in late gestation, hyperglycemia causes a time-dependent skeletal muscle Glut-1 drop, as is the case for Glut-4. Thus, there is a decrease in the skeletal muscle Glut-4 level with emerging insulin resistance.

The question that must then be answered is whether insulin has any effect on the fetus. In the rat model, insulin was administered to a 20-day-old fetus, a 2-day-old newborn, and a 60-day-old rat. A fourfold increase in the plasma insulin level was found; however, there was a concomitant 50 percent decrease in plasma glucose levels. Insulin therapy in the fetus appeared to increase the Glut-1 levels on a short-term basis, bringing it back to the baseline level. Glut-4 levels in the fetus and the newborn showed no difference across the board except for a slight decline at 60 minutes in the fetal muscle.

In humans, adults have shown an increase in insulin sensitivity with increased skeletal muscle Glut-4 levels, with enhanced translocation of Glut-4. In the fetus and the newborn it appears that there is no change from that in adults in the skeletal muscle Glut-4 level, and there is no effect on translocation of Glut-4. So, in comparison with published reports in which it has been described that adults on glucocorticoid therapy have developed insulin resistance (with a decline in skeletal muscle Glut-4 levels and a diminished translocation of Glut-4), the opposite occurs in the newborn. Thus, the effect of glucocorticoids on newborn Glut-4 translocation remains to be studied.

FORMULATION

Presented by Emmett Clemente, Ph.D.
*Chairman and Founder, Ascent Pediatrics, Inc.,
Wilimington, Massachussetts*

There is a $3.7 billion market for pediatric medications, compared with an estimated total $94 billion prescription market for both pediatric and adult therapeutic categories. As a comparison, neurologic products for the adult market are approximately $7 billion, twice the entire market for pediatric medications. The largest therapeutic category in pediatric medicine is antibiotics. Anti-infectives (antibiotics) make up 30 percent of the entire market for pediatric medications (Table 3-1). These data illustrate some of the reasons why large pharmaceutical companies have difficulty in developing pharmaceutical products for the pediatric patient: the therapeutic categories are many and market sizes are small compared to those for the adult market. To achieve an economic return, large companies would have to develop products across various therapeutic categories and enter the market with initial market potential which taken together is not feasible.

Factors that can increase the level of compliance and therefore improve the therapeutic outcome of medications in the pediatric population include dosing flexibility and dose administration. For example, most intranasal products being used for children are not specifically designed for the pediatric patient. Similarly, the volume of intraoccular medications are dosed on the basis of that for the adult eye, which can cause discomfort in the child. Palatability and appropriate dosage forms of oral medications are also important. For instance, it has been reported that up to 50 percent of children on oral steroids refuse to take their medicine because of the bitterness associated with these compounds. Because some of the alkaloids are very insoluble, their bitter taste is difficult to mask. Formulations that reduce dosing frequency are also needed.

TABLE 3-1 Important Pediatric Therapeutic Categories

Category	Class of Compound	Value of Category ($MM)
Anti-infectives	Antibiotic	$1,398
Cough/cold/allergy	Antihistamine/decongestant	385
Neurological	CNS stimulants/anticonvuls-ants	348
Respiratory	Bronchodilators	261
Dermatological	Topical	260
Anti-inflammatories	Steroids	249
Gastrointestinal	Antispasmodis	139
Analgesics	Antipyretic/analgesic	120
Hormones	Various	86
Ophthalmics	Topical	64
Antifungal	Fungicides	60
Subtotal		3,370
All other		334
Total		$3,704

SOURCE: Scott-Levin, Pharmacy Acquisition Dollars, 1997. Ascent Pediatrics, Inc., Wilimington, Mass.

Thyroxin is a compound with a very narrow therapeutic index. The present oral formulations include about 12 different dosage forms for the adult and the child. A neonatal patient with a nonfunctioning thyroid is administered thyroxin as a crushed tablet given in milk or water. There is no reliable way of knowing immediately that the infant has received an adequate dose. As the infant gets older, and because this compound is administered on a per kilogram basis, the accurate dosing of the child would be extremely difficult to accomplish with the present formulations. Instead, companies would need to formulate five to seven different dosage forms to accurately provide the medication to those children from birth to 6 years of age. In order to provide these formulations to the patient, formal regulatory approval is required (NDA) which includes acceptable chemistry manufacturing and control (CMC) data, as well as comparative clinical trials to demonstrate efficacy. The estimated market for this activity is between $3 million and $8 million a year, with product development time estimated to be between 5 to 7 years. These returns pose risks and returns that large companies are unwilling to undertake.

ANTI-INFECTIVES

Presented by Charles H. Ballow, Pharm.D.
*Director, Anti-Infective Research,
Kaleida Health Millard Fillmore Hospital*

The last 10 years has been an interesting time for anti-infectives development, with the decrease in the rate at which new, unique anti-infectives were being developed occurring at the same time as an increase in the bacterial resistance rate, especially among common pathogens, including those in the pediatric population. These factors have resulted in a resurgence of interest in the development of novel compounds for the treatment of infectious diseases.

During this time ongoing research has focused on the pharmacokinetics and pharmacodynamics of anti-infectives, and has been aimed at measuring the outcome from administration of an anti-infective. Two commonly studied measures of outcome are microbiologic cure and clinical cure. An additional goal of this research has been to link dosing and concentration in serum profiles with these outcome measures. In addition, recently published data demonstrate reduced resistance development when adequate serum concentrations are achieved (Thomas et al., 1998).

The primary reason for developing new techniques for studying the pharmacokinetics and pharmacodynamics of anti-infective agents revolves around an attempt to maximize patient outcomes while minimizing toxicity. When fixed-dose strategies are used for the administration of anti-infectives, the doses will often be too high or too low for some percentage of the population, perhaps even a third of the patients, because of either age, physiologic characteristics, or bacteriologic factors. Moreover, when fixed-dose profiles and clinical cure are used as endpoints, it necessitates the use of large patient databases to demonstrate efficacy and safety. Differences between and within drug classes complicate the study of the pharmacokinetics and pharmacodynamics of anti-infective agents. The site and type of infection and the population at risk must also be considered. The primary measure of bacterial susceptibility is the minimum inhibitory concentration (MIC). Three pharmacokinetic variables are commonly evaluated relative to the MIC. These are the ratio of the maximal concentration in serum (CMAX) to the MIC (CMAX/MIC), the time that the concentrations in serum exceed the MIC (T>MIC), and the ratio of the area under the curve (AUC) to the MIC (AUC/MIC or AUIC). These parameters are useful in understanding differences in microbiologic and clinical cure between drugs, not only in terms of the extent of cure but also in terms of the cure rate. These variables can be used to determine desirable concentrations for therapy. Thus, if concentrations are too low, the percent probability of microbiologic cure will be low. If the concentrations are too high, then the patient is exposed to higher concentrations of an anti-infective agent than necessary.

In a study of patients in an intensive care unit with nosocomial pneumonia, investigators demonstrated that the rate and extent of microbiologic cure were greater when the AUICs were higher than 125 (Forrest et al., 1993). There was a further increase when the AUICs exceeded 250. The likelihood of clinical cure was also greater with higher AUICs. Thus, there are advantages in linking pharmacokinetics with pharmacodynamics in terms of the rate and extent of bacterial killing because they translate into advantages in terms of clinical cure.

Chronic bronchitis serves as another example of a lower respiratory tract model useful for performing pharmacokinetic and pharmacodynamic analyses. In a recently conducted study, patients whose cultures tested positive for Haemophilus species were administered one of two regimens for 10 days: grepafloxacin at 400 milligrams once daily or clarithromycin at 500 milligrams twice daily. Samples for pharmacokinetic studies were collected after administration of the first dose and at steady state and serial sputum cultures were taken four times on the first day of dosing and then daily for nearly 14 days (Tran et al., in press). The rate and extent of bacterial eradication differed between the two anti-infectives with grepafloxacin having a greater extent and more rapid rate of eradication. Analysis of the pharmacokinetic and pharmacodynamic variables demonstrated a much higher AUIC for grepafloxacin compared with that for clarithromycin.

Relationships between the pharmacokinetics and pharmacodynamics of anti-infective agents can be used to predict what doses an individual patient needs to maximize the likelihood of cure while minimizing the risk of toxicity.
A limited number of studies in this area have been conducted with pediatric populations. The best work with pediatric populations has addressed otitis media. A retrospective pharmacokinetic-pharmacodynamic analysis conducted by Craig and Andes (1996) assessed microbiologic cure versus the time above the MIC for a number of anti-infective agents. A relationship was identified for both *Streptococcus pneumoniae* and *H influenzae* between eradication and $T>$MIC. When the concentrations in serum exceeded the MIC for greater than 40 percent of the dosing interval, maximal bacterial eradication was achieved. Moreover, as concentrations in middle ear fluid increased relative to the MIC, there was a nearly 100 percent likelihood of eradication.

Most of the studies of the pharmacokinetics of drugs in pediatric populations have used conventional dosing strategies, which presents a challenge because of the need to obtain multiple blood samples. Optimal sampling strategies (OSS) use applied statistical theory to identify a minimal number of key time points for drawing serum concentrations to provide the same information available by a conventional sampling design. Use of OSS may facilitate pharmacokinetic-pharmacodynamic research by making the conduct of such studies in pediatrics more feasible.

CHILDHOOD ASTHMA

Presented by Stanley J. Szefler, M.D.
Helen Wohlberg and Henry Lambert Chair in Pharmacokinetics and Director of Clinical Pharmacology, National Jewish Medical and Research Center, and Professor of Pediatrics and Pharmacology, University of Colorado Health Sciences Center

Asthma can occur early in life. Current therapy, even for children, is based on the concept that chronic inflammation is a key feature of asthma, but there is very little information on the time of onset of inflammation or the mechanism for its initiation, progression, and persistence. There is a general feeling among asthma care specialists that early childhood asthma is underdiagnosed and undertreated.

Current knowledge allows us to identify patients at high risk for asthma morbidity and mortality. Information is now developing regarding patients at risk for asthma, such as parental asthma, maternal smoking, atopic features and the presence of relevant allergens in the environment, and small lungs (National Heart, Lung, and Blood Institute, 1995, 1997). One of the consequences of undertreatment may be a loss over time of pulmonary function [FEV1] that is greater than that observed in patients without asthma and that is similar to that observed in patients with chronic obstructive pulmonary disease and cystic fibrosis (Lange et al., 1998; Peat et al., 1998; Weiss et al., 1995).

It is apparent that inhaled glucocorticoids are effective in controlling the symptoms of asthma and reducing the intensity of the inflammatory response in studies conducted with adults with asthma. This effect lasts as long as the treatment continues. No known treatment can consistently induce a lasting remission of the disease, and inhaled glucocorticoids have a relatively slow offset of effect compared with those of other long-term controller medications (Haahtela et al., 1994). Understanding the onset and progression of the inflammation, as well as its persistence, could provide insight into defining appropriate strategies for treatment depending on the stage of the disease (Peat et al., 1998).

Theories that early intervention with inhaled glucocorticoid therapy can be effective in preventing the progression of the disease and the risk for irreversible changes in the airways that could result in the persistence of symptoms have been developed (Agertoft and Pedersen et al., 1994; Haahtela et al., 1994; Overbeek et al., 1996; Selroos et al., 1995). Thus, there appears to be an effective opportunity for intervention.

Patients with "difficult to control asthma" have evidence of persistent inflammation (Lee et al., 1996; Leung et al., 1995; Wenzel et al., 1997). Their disease often has its onset in early childhood. Does this information suggest that children who manifest persistent inflammation despite anti-inflammatory therapy are at increased risk for disease progression? If so, it will be important to recognize these patients and provide more effective interventions at critical stages of their disease progression.

Gaps in Knowledge

Several key questions must be answered in developing treatments for asthma:

- If asthma is inflammation-based, when does the onset of inflammation take place?
- What cellular mechanisms are critical in the onset of inflammation? Are they the same mechanisms that allow progression of the disease? Is there a time when the disease is apparently out of control and not dependent on allergen stimulation? If so, what therapeutic interventions are appropriate for each stage of the disease? What is the role of the antigen-presenting cell in the pathophysiology of asthma? Is this cell affected by glucocorticoid therapy?
- Is there a "window of opportunity" for intervention? If so, what is the appropriate medication or combination of medications? What is the appropriate time for intervention? What criteria should be used for the initiation, titration, and discontinuation of treatment?
- Are inhaled glucocorticoids the drug of choice in managing the progression of early-onset childhood asthma? If so, do they affect long-term outcome? What are the risks-benefits involved in this treatment selection? What is the appropriate dose and method of administration?
- What are appropriate outcome measures that indicate progression of the disease? Are there reliable measures of pulmonary function and markers of inflammation that could be incorporated into clinical studies on early interventions in childhood asthma? Is FEV1 an adequate measure for monitoring disease progression? How does one account for the treatment effect on measures of pulmonary function?

A recent meeting of the FDA's Pulmonary and Allergy Drug and Endocrinology Advisory Panels concluded that the limits of safe and effective doses of inhaled glucocorticoids for children have not been defined (FDA, 1998a). Moreover, insufficient information is available on the long-term effects of asthma medications, especially inhaled glucocorticoids and leukotriene modifiers, administered to children at an early age and for prolonged periods of time.

Existing Recommendations for Stepwise Therapy in Adults and Children over Age 5

In recent guidelines asthma is classified as mild intermittent, mild persistent, moderate persistent, and severe persistent on the basis of symptoms and pulmonary function. A synopsis of recent guidelines suggests the following approach to asthma management in older children and adults (National Heart, Lung, and Blood Institute, 1995, 1997):

Intermittent: characterized as episodic bronchospasm. Therapy includes as needed ß-adrenergic agonists for the relief of symptoms. One can also prevent symptoms by administering a ß-adrenergic agonist before exercise or cromolyn–nedocromil before anticipated exposure to allergen.

Mild persistent: characterized by frequent episodes of bronchospasm, for example, more than twice per week but less than once per day, with marginal compromise in pulmonary function. First-line therapy may begin with an inhaled glucocorticoid (low dose),[*] cromolyn, nedocromil, or alternatively, sustained-release theophylline or a leukotriene synthesis inhibitor (zileuton [Zyflo–Abbott]) or antagonist (zafirlukast [Accolate; Zeneca]; montelukast [Singulair; Merck]). Medications can be combined to obtain beneficial effect. The doses of inhaled glucocorticoids may be increased if necessary. Inhaled ß-adrenergic agonists are used as needed for breakthrough symptoms.

Moderate persistent: characterized by daily symptoms, exacerbations that affect activity and sleep, and compromised pulmonary function. Inhaled glucocorticoids (medium dose)[*] are the cornerstone of treatment. A long-acting bronchodilator can be used for nighttime symptoms including a long-acting inhaled ß2-agonist (salmeterol), sustained-release theophylline, or long-acting oral ß2-agonist.

Severe asthma: characterized by frequent symptoms, exercise-induced asthma, nocturnal exacerbations, deterioration in pulmonary function, and compromised lifestyle. Inhaled glucocorticoids at higher doses are primary therapy. Other medications are added on the basis of need, for example, a long-acting ß-adrenergic agonist (salmeterol) or theophylline therapy to control night time symptoms and to prevent intermittent breakthrough. Short-acting ß-adrenergic agonists (albuterol, terbutaline, pirbuterol) are used to relieve breakthrough symptoms. Nedocromil may be included in an attempt to minimize the inhaled and oral glucocorticoid dose. Oral glucocorticoids are used for severe exacerbations and are occasionally needed as maintenance therapy. Once control is established, medications are reduced in a reverse order beginning with oral glucocorticoids, then as-needed ß-adrenergic agonists, followed by theophylline.

---

[*]In the National Asthma Education and Prevention Program Expert Panel Report II: *Guidelines for the Diagnosis and Management of Asthma,* doses of inhaled corticosteroids are classified as low, medium, and high and guidelines for the use of individual inhaled corticosteroids are provided (National Heart, Lung, and Blood Institute, 1997).

Stepwise Approach for Managing Infants and Children Under Age 5 with Chronic Asthma Symptoms

In younger children, the same classification system described above is used, but it is primarily based on symptoms, since pulmonary function is difficult to measure in young children. The following medications scheme is proposed in the National Asthma Education and Prevention Program guidelines (National Heart, Lung, and Blood Institute, 1997):

Intermittent: as-needed short-acting ß-adrenergic agonists to relieve symptoms. Short-acting ß-agonists are administered by a nebulizer or face mask and a spacer-holding chamber or oral liquid.

Mild persistent: first-line therapy may begin with cromolyn or nedocromil or low-dose inhaled glucocorticoid with a spacer-holding chamber and a face mask.

Moderate persistent: medium dose of inhaled glucocorticoids or, once control is established, medium dose of inhaled glucocorticoids and nedocromil or a long-acting bronchodilator (theophylline).

Severe asthma: high dose of inhaled glucocorticoids. If needed, add a systemic glucocorticoid at 2 mg/kg/day and reduce the dose to the lowest dose daily or alternate day that stabilizes symptoms.

Present Status of Inhaled Glucocorticoids as Cornerstone of Asthma Therapy

Numerous studies have shown that inhaled glucocorticoids improve asthma management and reduce inflammation in the airways. The response to inhaled glucocorticoids varies among patients. Recent observations suggest that the response to inhaled glucocorticoids is highly dependent on the time of intervention and that the earlier they are used the better (Agertoft and Pedersen et al., 1994; Haahtela et al., 1994; Overbeek et al., 1996; Selroos et al., 1995). The response to inhaled glucocorticoids is parameter specific, for example, a low dose may be effective in improving pulmonary function whereas a higher dose may be necessary to improve airway hyperresponsiveness (Pedersen and Hansen, 1995).

A high-dose, high-potency inhaled glucocorticoid (fluticasone propionate) or the use of delivery devices that improve drug delivery to the lung (budesonide with Turbuhaler) may be effective in improving pulmonary function and reducing the oral glucocorticoid requirement for patients with severe persistent asthma (Nelson et al., 1998; Noonan et al. 1995). Several recent studies have suggested that high-dose or long-term use of inhaled glucocorticoids may be associated with a higher risk for ocular disorders, such as glaucoma or cataracts (Cumming et al., 1997; Garbe et al., 1997, 1998).

There is no practical measure of airway inflammation for clinical application; therefore, clinicians must rely on symptoms and pulmonary function to guide therapy. The best pulmonary function measure for long-term follow-up appears to be FEV1. Additional pulmonary function measures could include FEV1 and forced vital capacity ratio, morning peak flow, and peak flow variation. The effect of ongoing therapy needs to be considered in the interpretation.

In general, long-term nonsteroid controller medications (for example, theophylline, leukotriene modifiers, long-acting ß2-agonists, cromolyn, and nedocromil) relieve and even prevent symptoms and also improve pulmonary function; however, their effect on long-term control of airway inflammation and disease progression is not clear. It is therefore difficult to adjust the inhaled glucocorticoid dose when indirect measures of inflammation, such as pulmonary function, can be ablated by nonsteroid long-term controllers.

Leukotriene Modifiers: An Attractive Alternative to Inhaled Glucocorticoids

Leukotrienes have been recognized as potent mediators of inflammation released by a number of cells involved in the inflammatory response to an allergic stimulus, namely, mast cells, basophils, eosinophils, neutrophils, and macrophages, all of which are present in the airways of patients with asthma. Leukotrienes are produced by the 5-lipoxygenase pathway of arachidonic acid metabolism and mediate bronchoconstriction and inflammatory changes important in the pathophysiology of asthma, such as the permeability of the microvasculature, mucus secretion, and neutrophil recruitment, and may contribute to airway edema.

In 1996, two medications in the leukotriene modifier class were approved for use in the treatment of asthma in the United States: zileuton, a 5-lipoxygenase enzyme inhibitor, and zafirlukast, a specific LTD4 receptor antagonist. In addition, another LTD4 receptor, antagonist, montelukast, was approved in 1998 by the FDA. The advantage of montelukast over the previous two medications in this class is that studies conducted with children as young as 6 years of age demonstrated efficacy (Kemp et al., 1998; Knorr et al., 1998) and were completed in children with asthma as young as 2 years of age. This has implications for application of this drug to the treatment of asthma in young children. In general, the medications in this class have the following properties:

1. immediate bronchodilator effect, as demonstrated by improvement in FEV1 by 10 to 15 percent over the baseline FEV1;
2. reduction of as-needed bronchodilator use by approximately 33 percent/day;

3. with chronic administration improvement in FEVI by approximately 10 percent over time;
4. reduction in nocturnal symptoms;
5. reduction in acute exacerbations requiring rescue medication;
6. ability to reduce inhaled glucocorticoid dose;
7. additive effect with inhaled glucocorticoid therapy;
8. additive effect with inhaled ß-adrenergic agonist effect;
9. reduced cellular inflammatory response to an inhaled allergen challenge in a sensitized patient;
10. reduction in blood eosinophil count demonstrated for zileuton and montelukast, suggesting a reduced chronic inflammatory response;
11. improved exercise tolerance demonstrated with single-dose (zafirlukast) and chronic (montelukast) therapy. (The latter observation suggests a reduction in airway hyperresponsiveness with chronic therapy);
12. efficacy in blocking pulmonary response to aspirin in aspirin-sensitive patients; and
13. no indication of tolerance or tachyphylaxis to the medication with chronic administration.

Leukotriene Modifiers: Classes Within a Class of New Medications

As noted earlier, there are two subclasses of medications within the class of leukotriene modifiers: the leukotriene synthesis inhibitors and the specific leukotriene receptor antagonists. These medications differ not only in their pharmacologic activities but also in their dosage schedules, susceptibilities to drug and food interactions, and indications for use in children of various ages.

Potential Applications of Leukotriene Modifiers

The leukotriene modifiers are an interesting new class of medications that have the benefits of oral administration. This is especially useful for children in whom administration of inhaled medications may present a difficulty. These medications have various potential applications: (1) they may be used as an alternative to inhaled glucocorticoid therapy in patients with mild persistent asthma who are unable to take inhaled medication; (2) they may be used as a supplement to inhaled controller medications to reduce the need for-high dose inhaled glucocorticoid therapy; (3) a medication with a different mechanism of action could have an additive effect with other medications in improving the overall response to treatment; (4) they could be seen as a potential benefit in the management of asthma patients who are sensitive to aspirin; and (5) they may offer the opportunity to individualize the approach to therapy as the differences in asthma pathophysiology among patients begin to be understood.

Current Areas of Interest in Childhood Asthma and Opportunities for Drug Development

To date, studies have not shown a reduction in the inflammatory response in the airways as a result of chronic therapy with leukotriene modifiers, especially in patients with moderate persistent or severe persistent asthma. In addition, studies have not shown reductions in collagen and tenascin deposition with chronic leukotriene moderator therapy, as previously reported with inhaled glucocorticoid therapy (Laitinen et al., 1997; Olivierie et al., 1997). One unique property of inhaled glucocorticoids is the relatively slow offset of the effect in pulmonary function control and airway hyperesponsiveness, especially after long-term therapy. This observation suggests that inhaled glucocorticoids have provided some long-term effects on the airways. To date, most of the studies with leukotriene modifiers have been short term, for example, 3 months, and they have not carefully evaluated the offset of the effect.

One of the more carefully studied leukotriene modifiers in relation to the resolution of airway inflammation have been pranlukast, a leukotriene antagonist. Of interest is the effect of this medication on maintaining asthma control and a number of markers of inflammation while reducing the inhaled steroid dose (Tamaoki et al., 1997), as well as the alteration of airway hyperresponsiveness (Hamilton et al., 1998) and a reduction of inflammatory cell numbers with chronic therapy (Nakamura et al., 1998a). Similar studies should be conducted with the other available leukotriene modifiers since the medications within this class may have different effects. Studies are also needed to demonstrate whether leukotriene modifiers have an effect on other allergic disorders, such as rhinitis, atopic dermatitis, conjunctivitis, and potentially, sinusitis and otitis. This would add another favorable dimension to this class of medications.

It has also been suggested that the response to these agents has been highly individualized, with some patients showing an excellent response and others showing no change in response. In general, it should be clear whether a patient is a responder or nonresponder within 2 weeks of treatment. It will be important to determine whether any difference in clinical response to these medications is related to genetic differences in the 5-lipoxygenase gene.

An understanding of the natural history of asthma would be helpful in establishing criteria for early diagnosis. Evaluation of the progressive aspects of the disease would be useful in defining appropriate measures of progression. The following areas deserve study: (1) establishment of the safety of various medications used as long-term controllers, specifically in relation to inhaled steroids and leukotriene modifiers; and (2) determination of the efficacies of certain medications in young children, including cromolyn, nedocromil, leukotriene modifiers, and inhaled steroids. For the available inhaled steroids and the respective delivery devices, research is needed to define the maximally safe doses and the minimally effective doses for various age groups and various levels of severity.

Drug research and development is needed in the following areas:

- dosage refinement for various drugs used in childhood asthma, especially for early intervention;
- identification of surrogate markers for medication evaluation;
- improved assessment of delivery systems;
- pharmacogenetics; and
- refined evaluation of drug metabolism and considerations of the efficacy and safety of inhaled glucocorticoids and the leukotriene modifiers.

Conclusions

Until proven otherwise, it appears that inhaled glucocorticoids are indeed the cornerstone of management for patients with moderate and severe persistent asthma. This is related to their proven effect on asthma control and their effect on resolving various measures of airway inflammation.

Leukotriene modifiers improve many measures of asthma control; however, except for pranlukast, there is limited information on their effect on resolving persistent airway inflammation. Studies are needed to determine whether the use of leukotriene modifiers alters the course of persistent asthma in a way that is comparable to that demonstrated with inhaled glucocorticoids. The role of leukotriene modifiers in mediating the course of asthma in children must be defined. Available data suggest that intervention with inhaled glucocorticoids, specifically, budesonide, has the potential to prevent the loss of pulmonary function. More studies with inhaled glucocorticoids are needed to verify this observation and to obtain comparable information for all long-term controllers.

Studies are needed to evaluate the safety of inhaled glucocorticoids with long-term treatment, considering the fact that they are now being suggested for use in young children. It must be recognized that the present concepts of treatment incorporate an earlier time of intervention and long-term treatment. Inhaled glucocorticoids with higher levels of potency (fluticasone propionate), better glucocorticoid delivery systems (Turbuhaler and hydro-fluoroalkane (HFA) propellant), and glucocorticoids that can be administered to very young children (nebulized budesonide) are now or will soon be available. As suggested by the FDA Pulmonary and Allergy Drug and Endocrinology Advisory Panels, it is important to define minimally effective and acceptably safe doses for the available inhaled glucocorticoids for various age groups including young children.

The minimal criteria for intervention with long-term therapy must be evaluated. Specifically, is the presentation of symptoms more than twice per week really an indicator for intervention with long-term controller therapy? A careful evaluation of surrogate markers and, possibly, biomarkers should be conducted to define drug efficacy in young children, as should short-term evaluation strategies that would reliably predict long-term effects.

PEDIATRIC ONCOLOGY

Presented by David G. Poplack, M.D.
*Elise C. Young Professor of Pediatric Oncology and
Head, Hematology Oncology Section, Department of Pediatrics,
Baylor College of Medicine and Director, Texas Children's Cancer Center*

Some 8,700 new cases of childhood cancer are diagnosed annually in the United States. Pediatric cancer is the leading cause of non-accidental deaths in children less than 15 years of age. The incidence of childhood cancer increased 6 percent from the mid-1970s to the mid-1990s.

Childhood cancer differs from adult cancer in its histology, reflecting significant biological differences. In addition, carcinomas that are common in adults are rarely seen in childhood. Lifestyle-related cancers also are not normally observed in the pediatric population. Breast, lung, prostate, and colorectal cancers are the main forms of malignancies seen in adults. In contrast, acute leukemias and central nervous system tumors predominate in children. A variety of other solid tumors, including neuroblastoma, Wilms' tumor, and retinoblastoma are generally specific to children.

Over the years there has been dramatic improvement in the survival and prognosis of children with these diseases. In 1960 few children with cancer were actually cured. The current 5-year survival rate is approximately 75 percent. The mortality rate has decreased nearly 50 percent from the early 1970s to the mid- to late 1990s, and has continued to decrease in the 1990s. There has been improvement over the years even in those diseases that traditionally have been more refractory to therapy, such as neuroblastoma.

The successes with pediatric cancer treatments are the result of a highly organized national clinical trials effort that was initiated and supported by the National Cancer Institute (NCI) in the 1950s. At present, more than two-thirds of patients newly diagnosed with childhood cancer are enrolled in one or more NCI-sponsored clinical trials. Approximately 5,000 children enter treatment trials each year. The NCI has developed a consortium of approximately 40 institutions focused on conducting Phase 1 studies of new anti-cancer agents. More recently, a pediatric brain tumor consortium was formed to develop clinical studies focused on these particularly difficult cancers.

In many ways, pediatric cancer has served as a paradigm. A number of treatment concepts that are routinely applied in the treatment of adult malignancies actually evolved from developments in the treatment of pediatric malignancies. In addition, numerous drugs currently used to treat adult cancer were initially developed for the treatment of pediatric cancer. For example, many agents originally developed for the treatment of acute lymphoblastic leukemia are now being used routinely in the treatment of a variety of adult malignancies. Nonetheless, it is important to conduct separate clinical trials for children and adults because the pharmacokinetics and pharmacodynamics of several anti-cancer agents differ between children and adults. In addition, the degree of prior therapy is frequently different, with children being more heavily treated before going on new agent trials than adults. Hence, prior therapy affects drug tolerance in children more so than in adults. For these reasons, the MTD (maximally tolerated dose) for a particular drug in children may differ significantly from that in adults. Pediatric oncologists are best qualified to prioritize, design, and implement clinical trials for children with cancer.

One of the challenges in the field is the relatively small number of patients available for pediatric new agent trials. As treatments become more successful, there will be fewer patients who relapse. Thus, there are fewer patients available for new agent studies at a time when there are more novel compounds to be studied. In part for this reason, pediatric cancer drug development is not profitable and has become, in many cases, an industry stepchild. In addition, because of the small numbers of patients available, multi-institutional trials are required. Also, because of the small patient numbers, the selection of the appropriate agents to be studied becomes critically important. In this regard there need to be better approaches to preclinical drug assessment so that only the most promising agents are advanced for clinical evaluation. Furthermore, better pre-clinical screening approaches that are more predictive for pediatric malignancies and that are also appropriate for the evaluation of the many new molecular and biologic therapies should exist. Such screening should also incorporate drug resistance models. Traditionally, in vitro screening approaches have relied on a panel of human malignancies made up almost exclusively of adult malignancies. It is important that screening be conducted using pediatric tumor cell lines.

Another important issue is how to approach the myriad drug analogues currently available. Because of limited patient numbers, pediatric clinical studies should evaluate agents with novel mechanisms of action. Assessment of analogues should be pursued using pre-clinical and animal models. Wherever possible, their utility initially should be validated in adult trials.

As the face of cancer biology changes, cancer therapy is changing. With the identification of novel molecular targets, specific targeting of pediatric malignancies has become an exciting and realistic prospect. With increasing frequency in the future, clinicians are likely to be using agents developed to target molecular targets unique for a particular pediatric cancer but not necessarily relevant to adult cancers.

Phase 3 trials for pediatric cancer have also been influenced by the improvement in overall prognosis. Most Phase 3 pediatric cancer trials are randomized studies. Over the years, as therapy has dramatically improved, the number of patients required to demonstrate a statistically significant difference between a newer and a "best available" therapy has increased. For example, to statistically demonstrate the increased effectiveness of adding a new agent to an acute lymphocytic leukemia induction regimen, when the current remission induction rate is well over 90 percent, would take many hundreds of patients. . For some pediatric tumors, Phase 3 trials now may take as long as four years to complete. Compounding these challenges is the fact that many new agents are available, including a variety of biologics, cytokines, differentiating agents, monoclonal antibodies, molecular therapies, and gene therapy approaches.

A major concern is the paucity of adequately trained pediatric cancer pharmacologists. Currently, Phase 1 trials are done at approximately 50 centers throughout the United States. Only a handful of these centers have active pediatric cancer clinical pharmacology laboratories; even a smaller number are actually training individuals in cancer clinical pharmacology. In many cases the type of clinical pharmacology training given is not formalized and is not adequate for the variety of new, molecularly targeted agents that will require study in the future. The pediatric cancer pharmacologist in the 21st century must not only be trained in pediatric oncology and classical clinical pharmacology but should also have an appropriate grounding in molecular biology. Training of such individuals may be the greatest single challenge for the field.

4

Extrapolation of Safety and Efficacy Data to Children

Extrapolation to children of safety and efficacy data generated for adults requires careful attention to potentially important differences between these two populations. The safety of drugs, for instance, needs to be supported by appropriate research with the targeted age group. Some medications that are completely safe for adults may produce toxic effects in children. An assessment of pharmacokinetic-pharmacodynamic relationships, however, by use of a surrogate and comparison of those results with those for adults, may suffice as a basis for approval of the drug for use in the pediatric population or help determine the doses to be used in clinical trial.

Unlike drugs, the majority of which are for oral administration, the majority of therapeutic biologics are for parenteral use only. Thus, many of the formulation issues for biologics to be used in the pediatric population are similar to the formulation issues for parenteral drugs to be used in the adult population. Because of their distinctive properties, the use of biologics results in unique safety concerns that require different types of monitoring, such as for adventitious agents that occur as a result of treatment with the biologic, or for reactogenicity. There is some concern about therapeutic biologics because little is known about the long-term effects of treatment with such agents, especially their effects on developing children. Many questions about the evaluation of biologics in the pediatric population need to be addressed; no simple approach is available.

The requirements for the safety and efficacy of medical devices are different from those for the safety and efficacy of drugs and biologics. Not only can the size of a device pose engineering problems, but hormonal influences and the activity levels of patients also need to be factored into the design of devices. Obtaining approval for use of a device in the pediatric population is also not an easy undertaking; ample evidence indicating that it has been properly designed for children and that the safety and efficacy are demonstrated rather than presumed must be made available.

Special considerations must be exercised when extrapolating safety and efficacy data in adults to children in the areas of drugs, biologics, and medical devices. The summaries of the presentations that follow explore such issues, including when and how safety and efficacy data can be used for children.

SPECIAL CONSIDERATIONS FOR EVALUATING MEDICAL DEVICES IN INFANTS AND CHILDREN

Presented by David W. Feigal, Jr., M.D., M.P.H.
*Director, Center for Devices and Radiological Health,
U.S. Food and Drug Administration*

Nearly 8,000 manufacturers have medical devices registered with the U.S. Food and Drug Administration (FDA). Many of these are specifically designed for children. Examples include heart valves, fetal bladder stents, medical equipment for the neonate, and hydrocephalus shunts. There are also life-supporting and life-sustaining products such as ventilators, rate-responsive pacemakers, and hemodiaylsis machines. These devices often cannot just be devices adapted from adult use. Even something as simple as the change needed in the size of a catheter lumen changes the flow characteristics and may critically affect product performance. Children grow and implants such as heart valves and hip prostheses need to be designed to accommodate growth or be designed for replacement. Changes in the type and level of activity occur rapidly from infancy to adulthood; some devices need to be developed with consideration given to the hormonal and body size changes that rapidly occur at adolescence.

To gain approval for a device for children, there must be evidence that it is properly designed for children, as well as a demonstration of safety and effectiveness. In contrast to drugs, for which formulation changes and improved palatability might be sufficient to develop a pediatric formulation, developers of pediatric devices must be focused on the performance and controls needed to adapt a device for a pediatric patient. Recently, the FDA centers responsible for drugs and biologics reviewed their approved products to identify those with inadequate clinical information to support pediatric labeling and published a list calling for pediatric studies. Contemplating a similar task for devices is daunting. Even aside from the fact the nearly half of all newly marketed devices are exempt from premarket applications, 4,500 new devices are approved or cleared for marketing in the United States each year. A device-by-device approach is not likely to work; more promising are the incentives to develop new devices for children.

The Center for Devices and Radiological Health (CDRH) gives priority to applications for novel products and products which address unmet medical needs and special populations. CDRH encourages consultation on device trials protocols in children under investigational device exemptions (IDEs—the experimental device application comparable to the IND for drugs and biologics). One of the most important issues to discuss is the evidence that needs to be developed for marketing clearance or approval.

The evidence needed to establish the safety and effectiveness of devices is somewhat different from the evidence needed to establish the safety and effectiveness of drugs and biologics. Device evidence is graded appropriate to the level of risk, ranging from nonclinical product performance standards to rigorous clinical trials. Although there is more flexibility in the evidence needed for approval, there is more room for disagreement. A provision in the Food and Drug Administration Modernization Act (PL 105-115) establishes procedures to resolve disputes and provisions for meetings with FDA officials to arrive at agreed upon criteria, evidence and study end points that in the absence of major scientific developments will be adequate to establish the safety and efficacy of the product.

Another mechanism to meet special needs is the humanitarian device exemption (HDE). This mechanism requires that fewer than 4,000 patients could use the device each year. No evidence of device effectiveness is required for an HDE, although informed consent and Institutional Review Board (IRB) oversight is necessary. Unlike orphan drug approval, HDE approval does not confer marketing exclusivity, and, in general, the HDE is more analogous to a drug treatment-IND-with-cost recovery than an orphan drug approval.

Finally, CDRH has a radiological health program that affects children. The standards set for radiation-emitting products range from clinical to nonmedical consumer devices. One of the programs for assessing medical x-ray exposure is the Nationwide Evaluation of X-ray Trends (NEXT) program, which sets standards and collects data from a testing program that recently measured the exposure to children from pediatric chest x-rays.

In summary, while developing devices for children presents many of the same challenges as developing drugs and biologics for children, and the tools differ, the need and potential remain great.

DEFINING SURROGATE ENDPOINTS AND BIOMARKERS FOR DRUG ACTION IN TRIALS WITH PEDIATRIC SUBJECTS

Presented by Robert Temple, M.D.
Associate Director for Medical Policy,
Center for Drug Evaluation and Research,
U.S. Food and Drug Administration

It is not clear whether the use of biomarkers and surrogates in the pediatric population poses problems different from the potential problems resulting from their use in adults. The U.S. Congress, in writing FDAMA, specifically incorporated into the law a provision that FDA had introduced in 1992, called *accelerated approval*, which allowed the use of surrogate markers that were less than well established but that nonetheless had a reasonable likelihood of predicting clinical benefit. FDA defines a surrogate endpoint as "a laboratory measurement or physical sign that is used in therapeutic trials as a substitute for a clinically meaningful endpoint that is for a direct measure of how a patient feels, functions or survives and is expected to predict the effect of the therapy" (57 *Federal Register* 13234–13242, 1992).

There is a tension between the advantages and disadvantages of the use of surrogates. As a general matter, reliance on surrogates can be faster, cheaper, and more efficient than use of clinical endpoints, but surrogates do not measure the endpoint of real interest. An additional drawback is that reliance on a surrogate results in a much smaller amount of controlled safety data than would be obtained from a trial with a clinically relevant endpoint. In addition, many risks do not manifest their effects immediately in children, for whom the problems raised by abnormalities in childhood might not show up until adulthood; short-term trials with surrogates give no opportunity to discover such effects.

This idea of relying on a surrogate endpoint is not new, but past practices have sometimes been reconsidered. In the past, FDA approved drugs that lowered ventricular premature beat (VPB) rates and were believed to lead to symptomatic improvement. But concerns arose over the proarrhythmic effects of these agents, and, notably, after a heart attack antiarrhythmic drugs were found to be lethal in some settings; thus these drugs are not being approved even for symptomatic treatments without evidence that they do not decrease survival. The FDA also approves drugs that lower blood pressure or lipids without premarketing evidence of other effects. FDA sometimes approves drugs because they shrink tumors, especially in patients with refractory illness, even though the consequences for the patient's health or survival are unproven.

Even when FDA bases initial approval on surrogate effects, subsequent outcome studies are of interest and importance. Moreover, the labeling for the drug reflects what is known. For example, if FDA approves a drug that lowers cholesterol levels it is approved for lowering cholesterol levels, not for improving survival. If a company wants to have the drug approved for improving survival, it must prove that it does. Thus, FDA usually distinguishes between approval of a drug on the basis of a surrogate effects and giving it a further claim on the basis of a surrogate effects.

The accelerated approval rule promulgated in 1992 and incorporated into law in 1997 (U.S. Food and Drug Administration Modernization Act §112, 1997) is aimed at drugs that treat serious illnesses for which no good therapy is available; in such cases FDA is prepared to rely on less well-established surrogates. There is currently no regulatory definition of a "well-established surrogate." The definition of "the strength of evidence" needed for a surrogate to support accelerated approval is that the surrogate must be "reasonably likely, based on epidemiologic, pathophysiologic, and other kinds of evidence, to predict outcome" (57 *Federal Register* 58942–58960, 1992). Presumably, a well-established surrogate has stronger support than is sufficient to be "reasonably likely" to predict benefits. Furthermore, it should be appreciated that in clinical trials there are endpoints that are not surrogates because they represent a real clinical benefit, but they are also not the final goal of therapy. These have been called *intermediate endpoints*. For example, increased exercise tolerance in patients with heart failure or decreased symptoms of hyperglycemia in patients with diabetes are valuable clinical benefits, but in both groups of patients a decrease in the rate of morbidity is hoped for as the final endpoint.

The main problem with surrogate endpoints is that they may not predict the desired outcomes. There are two possible reasons for this. First, the relationship between the surrogate and clinical endpoint may not be the causal relationship that is presumed. For example, improved bone mineral density does not always lead to a lower fracture rate. Second, drugs have more than one effect, and the surrogate endpoint measures only the one that is thought to be desirable. The drug could have other effects that are adverse. An outcome trial gives the "sum" of all these effects, but a trial with a surrogate endpoint does not. Examples include diuretics, which lower blood pressure but which also lower potassium levels, probably leading to arrhythmics, and antiarrhythmics, which decrease ventricular heartbeat rates but which probably increase the incidence of ventricular tachycardia and, perhaps, asystole. The net effect (beneficial or adverse) may depend on the populations and the duration of treatment. There may be some cumulative adverse effects that will not be observed in a short period of time.

In a number of situations it would be desirable to know the long-term effects of treatments, both in children and in adults. This is the case for such conditions as chronic lung disease, asthma, various inflammatory diseases, attention deficit disorder, and depression and psychosis. In many of these cases, the drugs that are being used have significant cardiovascular and other effects.

With these concerns in mind, there are certain situations that tend to support reliance on a surrogate endpoint, including consistent epidemiology, existence of appropriate animal models, and adequate understanding of disease pathogenesis. There are also practical reasons for relying on surrogate endpoints, such as a lack of existing therapy for a serious disease or the difficulty in conducting an outcome study, particularly when the effect would be very delayed or when the event rate is low.

Even if one can conclude that a drug is likely to behave in children like it does in adults, there could still be a concern as to whether the concentration-response relationship is the same. If the drug is not toxic and the drug is generally given on the plateau part of the dose-response curve, dosing can initially rely on the adult dose-response curve, modified for size, with a requirement to collect resulting safety information. If a drug is potentially toxic, an effectiveness trial is needed to establish an appropriate dose. Assessment of pharmacokinetic and pharmacodynamic relationships by use of a surrogate and then comparison of those with the relationships for adults might suffice as a basis for approval or might at least help determine the doses to be used in a clinical trial.

PREDICTION OF LONG-TERM EFFECTS ON POSTNATAL BRAIN DEVELOPMENT

Presented by Mark Batshaw, M.D.
*Chair, Department of Pediatrics,
George Washington University Medical Center, and
Director, Children's Research Institute,
Children's National Medical Center*

Brain development occurs rapidly from early embryogenesis to beyond birth. Some development is completed before birth, such as proliferation, neurogenesis, migration, and some synaptic generation. Other aspects occur after birth; it is these areas that can be affected by drugs given to children.

The organization of the brain starts at about the fifth month of gestation and progresses through about the sixth year of childhood. This involves the outgrowth of neurons and of the dendritic and axonal spines, the development of synapses, and the selective elimination of neural processes, as well as the proliferation of the glial network. In early childhood, when synapses are forming, the use of drugs may have very subtle effects.

Commonly occurring disorders involving neuropsychologic and neurophysiologic abnormalities can serve as surrogates for what could happen to a typically developing child who is exposed to drugs. For example, disorders of myelination, which starts at birth and continues for the first 2 years of life, can be studied to determine the possible effects of certain drugs on myelination. In addition, animal models, such as the trisomy 16 mouse, or the "quaking mouse," can be used as models of abnormal neuronal organization and myelination.

Neuropsychologic measures can be used to study the subtle abnormalities that drugs may produce. Such measures might be neuroanatomical, such as neuroimaging by magnetic resonance imaging (MRI) or computed tomography (CT). Some are neurophysiological, such as positron emission tomography (PET), single-photon emission computed tomography (SPECT), and functional MRI. Cognitive testing and neurobehavioral measures can also be used, although caution is in order with full-scale intelligence quotation (IQ) scores because they can mask subtle neuropsychologic patterns of abnormality.

Functional neuroimaging can also be used. This has recently been done with learning disability, especially dyslexia, by using PET and functional MRI scanning. In this case, glucose utilization or blood flow in various brain regions can be observed. Studies have shown decreased activation, that is, less glucose utilization or blood flow, in the left temporal parietal cortex, and the superior temporal cortex during rhyming-directed phonologic awareness. In dyslexia, persons have difficulty understanding phonemes, an understanding that occurs primarily in this temporal parietal cortex region. When one performs functional neuroimaging with dyslexic children, the occipital region lights up normally, but the temporal parietal region does not. One might be able to, in a similar way, look at functional neuroimaging in children before and after they receive a drug that could have adverse effects.

In terms of IQ testing and neuropsychology, it is difficult to predict long-term outcome in younger children. One of the main reasons for this is that the best predictor of intelligence is language. In the first 2 years of life, language is not well developed. The most commonly used test for children under 2 years of age is the Bailey Scales of Infant Development II, which provides global developmental status. The Wechsler intelligence scales are the most commonly used intelligence tests for children ages 3 to 16 years. These tests have the ability to assess verbal and nonverbal skills, working memory, and processing skills. These tests also provide a way of looking for abnormalities in cognition caused by drugs.

Some neuropsychologic tests can help pinpoint abnormalities in a specific area of the brain. For example, the Stroop test looks for cognitive flexibility. Slow performance is associated with left hemisphere dysfunction and traumatic brain injury. The Wisconsin card sort test assesses frontal and prefrontal functioning. These tests reveal much more subtle abnormalities than would be found by simply performing IQ studies. Investigators developing therapies such as radiation to the brain or drugs that are going to affect biogenic amines or excitotoxins (e.g., glutamate and glycine) should consider the value of these tests for determination of long-term adverse effects. As an example, animal models could provide an indication that a particular drug may affect the cerebellum. Tests that assess cerebellar function in humans might be in order.

Adaptive skill assessment, that is, the flexibility of the person in terms of performing daily living skills, can also be done to determine if a medication is having an effect on the ability of the patient to care for himself and herself. These tests identify a pattern of functioning different from the neuropsychological pattern. In addition, a number of child behavior checklists look at behavioral functioning and child competency.

EVALUATING BIOLOGIC THERAPEUTICS IN PEDIATRIC CLINICAL TRIALS

Presented by Karen Weiss, M.D.
*Director, Division of Clinical Trial Design and Analysis,
Center for Biologics Evaluation and Research,
U.S. Food and Drug Administration*

The definition of a biologic, as set forth in the Public Health Service Act, is "any virus, serum, therapeutic serum, toxin, antitoxin, vaccine, blood, blood component or derivative, allergenic product or analogous product, or arsphenamine or its derivative, or any other trivalent organic arsenic compound applicable to the prevention, treatment or cure of diseases or injuries in man."[*] That definition does not fully express the diversity of therapeutic products currently regulated by the Center for Biologics Evaluation and Research (CBER). Examples of therapeutic biologics will be discussed below, as will some differences between drugs and biologics. It is worth noting that Section III of FDAMA addresses exclusivity as an incentive for conducting needed pediatric studies. However, that exclusivity applies only to products approved under Section 505 of the Food, Drugs, and Cosmetics (FD&C) Act. Since most biologics are licensed under the Public Health Service Act, they are excluded from the exclusivity provisions of FDAMA.

Some of the more "traditional" therapeutic biologics fall into the broad category of cytokines, including interferons and interleukins and the category of hematopoietic growth factors, including erythropoietins and the colony-stimulating factors. Another class of therapeutic biologics is the monoclonal antibodies. The first licensed monoclonal antibody was Orthoclone (OKT3), for the treatment of renal allograft rejection. More recently, CBER has licensed monoclonal antibodies for the prevention of renal allograft rejection, for the treatment of Crohn's disease, and for the treatment of certain cancers.

CBER also regulates cell-based therapies when the cells are manipulated (e.g., selected or expanded). One example of such a cell-based therapy is Carticel, which is autologous cartilage derived from an auricular biopsy specimen, expanded in culture and placed into defects of the femoral condyle. CBER also regulates cell-based therapeutics when cells are from xenogeneic sources (e.g., mesencephalic porcine cells under investigation for the treatment of Parkinson's

---

[*]Public Health Service Act 1902 (42 U.S.C. 262) Section 351(a).

disease). A relatively new field of clinical investigation is gene therapy. Examples of investigational gene therapies include an adenoviral vector containing the *cftr* (cystic fibrosis transmembrane regulator) gene for cystic fibrosis and plasmids containing fibroblast growth factor for the treatment of coronary artery disease. CBER also regulates organ transplantation when the organs come from xenogeneic sources and combination products when the primary mode of action is the cellular component (e.g., hepatocytes housed in filters for the treatment of hepatic failure and pancreatic islet cells in alginate capsules for the treatment of diabetes mellitus).

Biologics differ from drugs in important ways. One is that the starting or source material for many biologics is cellular or cell substrate in origin. Such products have the potential to transmit infectious agents. The manufacturing procedures must be sufficient to remove or inactivate infectious agents. Biologic licensing regulations call for strict controls over the entire manufacturing process to ensure, to the extent possible, that the biologic product is sterile, pure, and potent.

Another difference between biologics and drugs is that many therapeutic biologics are large proteins. Administration of foreign protein, particularly chronically, may result in an immune reaction. Although a serum immunologic response (i.e., a protective antibody) is the basis for the effectiveness of vaccines, the development of an immune response after exposure to a therapeutic biologic is not desirable. An immune response may simply manifest as an elevated serum antibody titer that has no clinical sequelae. At the other extreme it may result in unwanted effects such as altered pharmacokinetics, which could render a product ineffective, or it may manifest as serious or life-threatening anaphylaxis. The likelihood that an immune reaction will occur tends to be higher with repeated administration of a foreign protein, but such a reaction could even occur after single-dose administration. Information on serum antibody levels after exposure to the biologic and clinical aspects of immune reactions is among the important types of safety data that must be generated during clinical development. The detection of serum antibody formation requires a sensitive laboratory assay; if no assay is available, the sponsor needs to develop and validate an assay. This procedure may be costly and time-consuming.

The development of immune reactions from administration of a biologic also has implications in the design of studies with animals and the ability to use animal data to support human trials. Generally, for drug products, long-term dosing (e.g., 9 to 12 months) is a necessary prerequisite to chronic dosing in humans. However, nonhuman animals, including nonhuman primates, often develop neutralizing antibodies to biologics, sometimes after only a single exposure, making repeat dosing potentially impossible and irrelevant.

Unlike drugs, the majority of which are for oral administration, the vast majority of therapeutic biologics are for parenteral use only. Thus, many of the biological product formulation issues for pediatric populations are similar to the formulation issues for parenteral drugs: the safety and feasibility of different volumes and concentrations, the safety of various preservatives, the appropriate packaging of vials or prefilled syringes for pediatric use, and so forth.

There is no simple approach to the evaluation of a biologic product for use in the pediatric population. One needs to think about the intended action or the indication of the particular biologic and the disease or condition that it is proposed to treat. Questions that should be considered during development include the following: Is the disease unique or very common in the pediatric population? Are there alternative therapies? What are the safety and efficacy profiles of those alternative therapies that will make it imperative or important to develop a new agent? What is the relevance and suitability of the adult safety and efficacy data? Will it be possible to extrapolate efficacy data from older to younger children? The answers to these questions are among the considerations for optimizing the program development for biologics for the pediatric population.

The evaluation of the clinical efficacy of biologics is similar to that for drugs and devices. There may be unique safety concerns for biologic products because of their distinctive properties that will require different types of monitoring, such as for adventitious agents or for immune reactions. Little is known about the long-term effects (e.g., years) of treatment with therapeutic biologics, especially the effects on growing children. As more and more biologics are licensed for use for chronic treatment, it will be important to collect and examine data from postmarketing use, including studies from registries and Phase 4 clinical trials (controlled studies following market approval), to further the understanding of this important class of agents.

5

Raising Awareness of Regulatory, Legal, and Ethical Issues

Every year, information necessary for the proper use of drugs and biologics in infants and children is lacking for more than half of newly approved drugs and biologics that are likely to be used by children. This is often because children are not sufficiently included in research studies. Pediatric clinical trials involve many logistical challenges as well as legal and regulatory considerations. For instance, a special consideration is informed consent and whether parental consent, the assent of the child, or both are required.

The U.S. Food and Drug Administration's (FDA's) new Pediatric Rule makes it more likely that children will receive improved treatment, because physicians will have more complete information on how drugs affect children and the appropriate doses for each age group (FDA, 1998e). The rule also allows FDA to require industry to test already marketed products in studies with pediatric populations in certain compelling circumstances, such as when a drug is commonly prescribed for use in children but when the absence of adequate testing and labeling could pose significant risks. The intent of this session is to examine the many interrelated legal and regulatory issues, as well as the interrelated social and ethical concerns, in the evaluation of the effects of drugs and biologics on pediatric populations.

FDA PERSPECTIVE ON NEW REGULATIONS

Presented by Dianne Murphy, M.D.
*Associate Director for Pediatrics,
Center for Drug Evaluation and Research,
U.S. Food and Drug Administration*

In 1994, FDA provided a new regulatory approach to encourage studies with pediatric populations to develop information on the proper use of a product being prescribed for the pediatric population. With that regulatory approach, where appropriate, FDA could conclude that the course of the disease and the effects of a drug, both beneficial and adverse, were sufficiently similar in the pediatric and adult populations to permit extrapolation of efficacy in adults to efficacy in children. In such a situation, there would be no need to again prove efficacy in the pediatric population. Unfortunately, the rule did not achieve its intended objectives. Seventy-seven percent of the labeling changes proposed by drug companies in response to this rule did not result in improved labeling for children. To improve on that record, two additional legislative and regulatory tools are now available: (1) Section III of the 1997 Food and Drug Administration Modernization Act (FDAMA; PL 105–115), which provides 6 months of additional marketing exclusivity, and (2) the 1998 Pediatric Rule which requires studies in the pediatric population unless such studies are waived or deferred.

Under FDAMA, which is voluntary, the studies to be submitted by the sponsor must be responsive to a written request issued by FDA. The way in which this actually works is that the sponsor first submits a proposal of what studies it thinks will be necessary. FDA's written request in response to that proposal is based on its assessment of what studies are needed to produce a health benefit in the pediatric population. Having a sponsor submit a proposal first allows FDA to determine the level of interest in and commitment to pursuing studies for a particular moiety. Because the additional exclusivity will attach to the "active moiety," the sponsor may need to provide the results of studies for all products with that moiety if those products are being used in pediatrics but are not appropriately labeled for such use.

As of May 1999, of the 15 technical divisions in the FDA's Center for Drug Evaluation and Research, all but two had received proposals. As of May 23, 1999, there were 133 proposals and FDA had issued 83 written requests asking for 155 studies. Fifty-five of these studies were efficacy and safety studies, 55 were pharmacokinetic studies, and the remaining were pharmacokinetic or pharmacodynamic, safety only, or "other" types of studies. "Other" includes prophylaxis studies and studies of the actual use of over-the-counter products. During this period 14 studies were proposed for the neonatal population and 24 studies were proposed for the population less than 2 years old. Physiologic and functional childhood changes and development often occur across the arbitrary age groups defined in the 1994 regulation. Most of the requested studies reflect these fundamental realities and include subjects in a number of age ranges. FDA realizes the need for flexibility in this area and is basing requests on the needs of science and is not constrained by age groups.

Because FDAMA is voluntary and does not include biologics, old antibiotics, or products without remaining patents or exclusivity, the Pediatric Rule was published in December 1998. Compliance with the Pediatric Rule is not voluntary. Under the Pediatric Rule, applications for new drug approvals must include results of studies with the pediatric population unless FDA has waived or deferred these studies. FDA has, however, stated that it will *not* delay approval of a product for adults if the result of studies in the pediatric population are not ready. The driving principle behind the Pediatric Rule has been the generation of information with respect to: (a) those drugs that will provide meaningful therapeutic benefit (defined as a significant improvement in the treatment, diagnosis, or prevention of a disease); and (b) drugs for which there is a need for additional therapeutic options. These study requirements may be waived if the drug does not meet the criteria for meaningful therapeutic benefit and substantial use. Alternatively, these studies may be deferred if additional safety and effectiveness information is needed from the adult usage or if the product is ready for approval for adult use. The sponsor must, however, have a plan for such studies and must have obtained a deferral that states when the results of the studies are to be submitted. In summary, under the Pediatric Rule, at the time of approval, a new drug application must include studies in the pediatric population, a waiver for such studies, or an agreement on the deferral of pediatric studies.

FDA must report to the U.S. Congress on the impact of FDAMA's Pediatric Exclusivity by legislation by January 2001. In addition to determining the economic impact of the program and any suggestions for modification, the agency will focus on the types of studies that have been useful in providing needed information, endpoints that have been studied and proven to be useful, and the pharmacokinetic or pharmacodynamic approaches that can be used to decrease the need for efficacy studies in certain diseases.

ROLES OF INSTITUTIONAL REVIEW BOARDS AND DATA-MONITORING COMMITTEES IN CLINICAL TRIALS

Presented by Susan S. Ellenberg, Ph.D.
*Division of Biostatistics and Epidemiology,
Center for Biologics Evaluation and Research,
U.S. Food and Drug Administration*

Data-monitoring committees (DMCs) and institutional review boards (IRBs) serve different but complementary roles in clinical trials. The major responsibility of the IRB is to ensure that all research conducted in the institution for which it is responsible is appropriate and safe for the projected study population. Its review focuses on the initial design and study protocol, although IRBs do receive information about serious adverse effects in real time during the trial and are required to perform regular rereview of studies with whatever updated information is available to the study sponsor. The responsibility of the DMC, in contrast, focuses on the interim data accumulated as the trial progresses. An independent DMC will not necessarily be established for every clinical trial, but when one exists it is usually the only trial component that has access to the unblinded interim data. Thus, a DMC has primary responsibility for detailed consideration of the interim data and for recommending any changes (including early termination) in the study protocol. An IRB generally does not have either the time or the requisite expertise to perform such intensive interim reviews.

A DMC may be defined as a group of experts that reviews the ongoing conduct of a clinical trial to ensure continuing patient safety as well as the validity and scientific merit of the trial. These committees are also frequently referred to as data and safety monitoring boards, or by other similar designations. DMCs were first established as components of trials sponsored by the National Institutes of Health starting in the 1960s. In recent years, their use has expanded among federally sponsored trials and especially industry-sponsored trials.

Monitoring of ongoing clinical trials is important. Monitoring is needed to ensure that any unexpected safety concern is identified as rapidly as possible. Monitoring is also important to detect and correct problems in trial conduct, such as lagging accrual, unacceptably high ineligibility rates, lack of compliance with the study protocol, and excessive numbers of dropouts. Finally, monitoring allows for the possibility of early termination of the trial when the results are either so strongly positive or negative that the likelihood is small that the conclusions would change if the trial were to continue to its planned conclusion.

Typically, DMC members are physicians specializing in the disease being studied and biostatisticians with experience in the design and analysis of clinical trials. Frequently, DMCs will include a bioethicist, particularly when the trial is addressing a major public health issue or when the trial raises difficult ethical issues. Some trials will require other types of expertise for adequate monitoring—for example, basic science, pharmacology, epidemiology, and law. In some cases a patient advocate or community representative will be appointed as a committee member.

A variety of models have been proposed for DMC operations, and many different models are in use (Ellenberg et al., 1993). There is variation in the sizes of committees, the frequency and type (in-person or conference call) of meetings, attendance or participation of individuals other than committee members at meetings, formats for presentation of data to the DMC, and many other aspects of DMC operations. Although some differences may be explained by differences in the types of trials (highly complex trials addressing multiple questions may, for example, require a larger DMC than simpler studies with a single focus), other differences have been controversial (Fleming and DeMets, 1993; Meinert, 1998).

Although all clinical trials require monitoring, all trials do not necessarily need a formal DMC. DMCs are most important when the treatments address a major outcome—for example, in trials of potentially lifesaving treatments. In such trials, an unanticipated safety issue or a large treatment effect that appears early in the trial may raise ethical concerns about continuing the trial as designed. It is optimal when those scientists making judgments as to whether the interim data are strong enough to support reliable conclusions do not have financial, intellectual, or other ties to the study outcome that could inappropriately influence these judgments.

"Independent" DMCs include no representatives from the industry sponsor, the study investigators, or others with some vested interest (either financial or intellectual) in the outcome of the study. Independent committees help ensure the objectivity of decision making, as described above. In addition, they reduce the chance that the conduct of the study will be affected by the awareness of the interim data. For example, a study investigator with knowledge that the data are even slightly trending toward the superiority of one of the study treatments may cease to enter patients in the study, may begin entering only certain types of patients in the study, or may encourage or facilitate patient noncompliance and dropout (Green et al., 1987).

Despite their importance in clinical trials, DMCs have received little attention in the regulatory arena. Independent DMCs are not required for any trials except for the very limited subset of trials performed in emergency situations in which informed consent is waived (21 CFR [*Code of Federal Regulations*] 50.24). The purpose and operations of DMCs are briefly discussed in guidance documents on good clinical practices and on statistical principles for clinical trials (FDA, 1997a; 1998). Both of these documents emerged from the International Conference on Harmonization, a collaboration of industry and regulatory authorities in the United States, Europe, and Japan to optimize and standardize drug development practices and policies internationally.

DMCs have monitored many trials with pediatric populations in areas such as AIDS, cancer, and other serious diseases. In principle, there are no reasons why DMCs for pediatric studies would operate any differently from DMCs for adult studies except for the types of expertise that would be needed on the committee. The fact that ethical concerns may, on average, be more intense for trials with pediatric populations because children are a "vulnerable population" who cannot provide full informed consent for their treatment suggests, however, that DMCs may be particularly valuable for many trials with pediatric populations.

ETHICS OF DRUG AND BIOLOGIC RESEARCH IN INFANTS AND CHILDREN*

Presented by Robert M. Nelson, M.D., Ph.D.
*Associate Professor of Pediatrics and Bioethics,
Medical College of Wisconsin*

An individual child may benefit from participation in research in a variety of ways, including access to new therapeutic interventions or from close individual monitoring (Nelson, 1998). Although an alternative to participating in research is to receive the currently available treatment, the assumption that these treatments are safer and more effective than interventions under investigation may not be justified. In fact, most drugs used to treat children have never been tested formally, making off-label use of medications the de facto standard of care in pediatrics. It follows that inadequate information may expose children to unexpected adverse reactions or to suboptimal treatment. In addition, the lack of a pediatric formulation of a drug may deny a child access to an important therapeutic advance or expose a child to a drug in homemade, poorly absorbed preparations.

In other words, if children have not been sufficiently included in research, adequate information may be lacking to guide the pediatric use of a medication. Thus, any particular child may be exposed to greater risk and deprived of potential benefit compared with the risk and benefit for an adult, given the same medication, an unfair difference based solely on age. This situation may be due to regulatory impediments, economic disincentives, or reluctance to require studies with pediatric populations unless the primary use of a drug will be by children. Also, the logistics of performing research with pediatric populations may be more difficult given, for example, the lower incidence of a disease in children, the complexity of the developmental changes that may be taking place in children, and the limited market for the recapture of the costs of drug development.

The American Academy of Pediatrics (AAP) Committee on Drugs (1995) argues that drug researchers have an ethical obligation to conduct drug (and biologics) research with children:

> There is a moral imperative to formally study drugs in children so that they can enjoy equal access to existing as well as new therapeutic agents. . . . The AAP believes it is unethical to deny children appropriate access to existing and new therapeutic agents. It is the combined responsibility of the pediatric community, pharmaceutical industry, and regulatory agencies to conduct the necessary studies; it is the responsibility of the general public to support the necessary research in order to assure that all children have access to important medications and receive optimal drug therapy. (pp. 287, 294)

---

*Portions of the text were adapted from Nelson (1998).

This claim rests on two assertions:

1. Given the widespread "off-label" use of drugs and biologics by pediatricians, children are being harmed (either by the presence of adverse events or by absence of therapeutic effect) by the lack of basic safety and efficacy data concerning the pediatric use of a drug or biologic.
2. This "harm" can be reduced or eliminated through properly designed and conducted clinical studies of a drug or biologic with children as participants.

Although this claim is widely shared, it is difficult to estimate the exact nature and extent of the harms suffered by children in the absence of such information.

Four issues are important in considering the ethics of drug and biologics research with infants and children: (1) anchoring studies to "minimal risk," (2) current regulations guiding clinical research, (3) placebo-controlled trials, and (4) respecting a child's assent or dissent concerning participation in research.

Anchoring Studies to "Minimal Risk"

The dominant interpretation of the requirements of justice in research has been to protect so-called "vulnerable" populations from exposure to an inappropriate share of risk in the absence of certain benefit. One way to protect against the involuntary assumption of research risk is the requirement for obtaining voluntary and informed consent, a requirement that excludes persons who are incapable of providing informed consent (e.g., children and mentally disabled people) or who, if capable, may not be in a position to provide voluntary consent (e.g., prisoners). Although perhaps reasonable for adults, such a consent requirement would preclude all research with children who are not legally or developmentally capable of providing voluntary and informed consent. The inability of children to provide consent has led to restrictions based on the stratification of research proposals according to risk. The conceptual cornerstone of current research policy, the Belmont Report (National Commission, 1979), interprets the principles of respect for persons, beneficence, and justice as requiring the protection of children through limitation of the risk to which a child may be exposed regardless of parental permission. The concept of "minimal risk" serves to anchor allowable risk to the risk encountered in the normal course of a child's everyday life. The challenge to enhance justice in regard to pediatric research is to broaden the participation of children who are not capable of consent while at the same time minimizing any exposure to risk that may not be balanced by an appropriate benefit for that particular child, or for children with the condition being studied.

Current Regulations Guiding Clinical Research

Both investigators and institutional review boards familiar with clinical trials with children should assist in ensuring the use of practices (FDA, 1998b) that safeguard the child participant (American Academy of Pediatrics Committee on Drugs, 1995). Particular attention needs to be directed to the International Conference on Harmonization (ICH) guidance on good clinical practice, which contains a section (Section 4) on nontherapeutic trials with children (FDA, 1996). Population pharmacokinetic approaches may mitigate several of the problems associated with conducting pharmacokinetic studies with pediatric populations (FDA, 1998c).

All research involving human subjects conducted, supported, or otherwise subject to regulation by any federal department or agency is subject to the U. S. Department of Health and Human Services (DHHS) Policy for Protection of Human Research Subjects (45 CFR 46). The issues of consent and assent for pediatric patients enrolled in clinical trials are discussed in this DHHS regulation. If the study is performed under a U.S. investigational new drug application (IND), the informed consent (21 CFR 50) and IRB (21 CFR 56) regulations apply. If the study is not performed under a U.S. IND but the data are submitted as part of a new drug application, a biologics license application, or a product license application, the standards of the country in which the study is performed or the Declaration of Helsinki standards, whichever provides greater protection for the subjects of the study, must be met (21 CFR 312.120).

Placebo-Controlled Trials

Randomized controlled trials (whether they are against placebo or active treatment) may be necessary to be able to infer that an intervention (drug, biologic, or device) is effective for the selected population under the conditions of the study. The research imperative, to the extent that it privileges the knowledge gained from randomized controlled trials over clinical knowledge gained in the practice of medicine, may do a disservice to physicians and patients. However, the uncritical and anecdotal application of medical technology based on "biologic plausibility" or the uncontrolled "case series" experience of a group of physicians is also problematic.

FDA focuses the urgency or moral requirement to do research with the notion of "meaningful therapeutic benefit" (FDA, 1998c). Yet, how is "meaningful therapeutic benefit" to be determined? If no drug or biologic is approved for use by children with the indicated condition or disease (and no drug or biologic is, thus, labeled for this indication), a new entity will by default have a "meaningful therapeutic benefit" regardless of the efficacy of other "off-label"* treatments. The possibility of an "off-label" use of a drug that provides a "meaningful therapeutic benefit" appears to be disallowed in the absence of published data that establish the safety and effectiveness of that medication. Thus, the restricted comparison with labeled products in determining "meaningful therapeutic benefit" may undervalue "off-label" clinical knowledge and reinforce the apparent need for a placebo-controlled trial regardless of the medical standard of care.

Placebo-controlled trials are controversial, especially those with children. The argument about placebos centers on two general issues: (1) scientific necessity, and (2) ethical appropriateness. The question, then, is how this placebo controversy translates into the pediatric setting. When is a placebo control justified in research with children? This question can be addressed in two steps: (1) If efficacy has been established in adults, what further information is necessary to establish efficacy in children? (2) If it is necessary to establish efficacy in children in the absence of applicable data from adults, is a placebo-controlled trial necessary and justified (that is, ethical)? First, FDA allows for the possibility that the safety and effectiveness of an intervention for the pediatric population can be established on the basis of data for adults and appropriate pharmacokinetic data. Second, FDA acknowledges that a placebo-controlled trial may not be necessary. However, this admission is of limited value in getting away from the initial use of placebo controls. According to the FDA, only when there is an established effective treatment will it be unnecessary to perform further placebo-controlled trials. The crux of the problem lies in the determination of efficacy.

In the absence of an adequate and well-controlled study published in the medical literature, it is highly doubtful that FDA would accept a current "off-label" pediatric use of a biologic or drug as effective (absent pharmacokinetic data and study with adults establishing effectiveness). The results of an active-control equivalence trial, no matter how well designed, would not be accepted as evidence if neither of the treatments being compared had been studied against a placebo.

How, then, might an IRB evaluate design of the research that involves children and that includes a placebo-control arm? One specific issue in the IRB review of "placebo-controlled" trials is the analysis of benefit. Approval under Section 405 requires the "prospect of direct benefit." If the inclusion of a placebo-controlled arm is interpreted as not offering the prospect of direct benefit, the protocol can be approved only under Section 404 (if the research involves no greater than minimal risk) or Section 406 (if the research involves only a minor increase over minimal risk). Since research considered under Section 405 is not indexed to minimal risk but must simply be commensurate with the

---

*Off-label means the clinical use of a drug or device for an indication, using a dosage form or a dose regimen, for a patient population or other drug or device use parameter which is not mentioned in the approved label.

available alternatives, the determination of whether a protocol does or does not offer the prospect of direct benefit directly impacts on the allowable level of risk exposure (DHHS, 1983, 1991b). The controversy over the placebo-controlled trial of human growth hormone illustrates the important difference between what has been called a "prerandomization" analysis of benefit and a "postrandomization" analysis of benefit. In effect, for an IRB to decide that the placebo-control arm of a randomized trial does not have the prospect of direct benefit is to "prejudge precisely the information the research is designed to discover" (Williams, 1996).

The issue, then, is not the inclusion of a placebo arm but whether an effective treatment is being denied to those who are randomized to the placebo arm. If the medical standard of care involved an otherwise nonvalidated treatment but was nevertheless believed to be effective by the involved physicians (and other IRB consultants), an IRB would likely deny approval of the study on the basis of the potential of harm to the children in the placebo-control arm from being denied the standard "effective" treatment. Further justification would likely be needed (beyond the fact that the current standard treatment had never been evaluated against a placebo) to make the case that an IRB should approve the protocol.

Consent, Assent, and Determination of Risk

The Report and Recommendations on Research Involving Children of the National Commission for the Protection of Human Subjects of Biomedical and Behavioral Research (the National Commission) was published in 1977 and is the foundation for the 1983 federal regulations known as Subpart D of Title 45, *Code of Federal Regulations*, Part 46 (DHHS, 1991a). In addition, the National Commission also issued the Belmont Report on the basis of the ethical principles and general guidelines that ground the more specific rules governing research with human subjects. The Belmont Report identified three principles: (1) respect for the rights of the individual (on the basis of respect for persons), (2) the obligation to protect the individual from undue risk (beneficence), and (3) fairness in the distribution of the burdens and benefits of research (justice).

Subpart D, based on the National Commission's Report on Research Involving Children (National Commission, 1977), incorporates these added protections on the basis of a risk classification anchored to the concept of minimal risk. The concept of "minimal risk" was meant to serve as a limit to parental authority to enroll a child in "nontherapeutic" research.

The National Commission recognized that parents make day-to-day decisions that concern their children's medical treatment, and such decisions are based on a balancing of risks and benefits. The National Commission applies this discretionary authority of the parent to "therapeutic" research regardless of the absolute level of risk, provided that the risk is justified by the anticipated benefit to the child and that the relation of the anticipated benefit and risk is at least as favorable as those of the available alternative approaches. In fact, IRBs are explicitly advised to "evaluate [therapeutic] research protocols . . . in the same way that comparable decisions are made in clinical practice" (National Commission, 1977). Thus, for research that may directly benefit a child, the acceptability of risk is left to the discretion of the parent, provided that an IRB believes that the risks and benefits of the research project are comparable to those of the other available options, a condition that has been referred to as "clinical equipoise" (Freedman, 1987). Under such circumstances, the assent of the child or the permission of the parent is sufficient for participation in the research.

The National Commission then extends the scope of parental authority into research that offers no benefit to the child by comparing the child's research experiences with those that are normally encountered apart from being a research subject. Parents have the responsibility and authority "to choose activities and to define a manner of life for their children." The National Commission asserts that "many of the experiences which parents generally allow to their children are somewhat risky and cannot be said, without forcing the case, to involve particular benefits." Consequently, "when risks entailed in research are equivalent to normal risks of childhood, parents may properly permit these risks" (National Commission, 1977).

The National Commission assumes that parental discretion properly operates to balance the risks and benefits of everyday life. Nevertheless, the question of whether the risks and benefits of participating in research are similar to that of a child's nonresearch experiences is not left up to the sole discretion of a child's parents, apart from the limited situation in which the child may directly benefit from the research. With a definition of "minimal risk," the National Commission seeks to create a research environment that resembles this everyday context and thus to specify the limits of parental authority in permitting a child to participate in nonbeneficial research. "Minimal risk" is defined as "the probability and magnitude of physical or psychological harm that is normally encountered in the daily lives, or in the routine medical or psychological examination, of healthy children" (National Commission, 1979). Thus, the definition of "minimal risk" specifies the conditions under which parents may appropriately allow a child to participate in any activity, whether in the context of research or in the course of daily life. In effect, the scope of parental authority is extended to cover a child's participation in nonbeneficial research if the risks are reasonably commensurate with those of the child's nonresearch life. In doing so, the National Commission set up two further problems: first, should the risk that a child is exposed to vary depending on the child's particular life experience? and, second, does a parent have the authority to expose a child to any increased risk when there is no hope for benefit for that particular child?

The National Commission introduced the concept of "minimal risk" in an attempt to provide a boundary condition that serves to limit parental discretion to permit a child's participation in research. In effect, before allowing a parent to permit a child's participation in research, an IRB was to determine the extent to which the research presented a range of risks and benefits commensurate with that child's situation. The federal regulations define "minimal risk" as "the probability and magnitude of harm or discomfort anticipated in the research are not greater in and of themselves than those ordinarily encountered in daily life or during the performance of routine physical or psychological examinations or tests" (45 CFR 46.102(I)). This definition omits the phrase "of healthy children" that is found in the National Commission's report, creating an ambiguity that the risks of research may be indexed to the "ordinary" experiences of sick children rather than those of healthy children. The National Commission suggested four perspectives that need to be considered in estimating the allowable risk: common sense, the investigators' experiences, any statistical information, and, finally, the situation of the proposed subjects. The last perspective also raises the possibility that allowable risk will be indexed to the actual risks experienced by a particular child and does not indicate whether the risks should be evaluated from an adult's perspective or from a child's perspective.

The National Commission's decision to permit nonbeneficial research involving greater than minimal risk if the research investigated a child's "disorder or condition" presented the most controversy. The majority argument in favor of allowing children to participate in nonbeneficial research that presents greater than minimal risk was largely pragmatic. The National Commission noted that "parental authority routinely covers a child's participation in many activities [such as skiing and contact sports] in which risk is more than minimal, and yet benefit is questionable." They were also "impressed by reported examples of diagnostic, therapeutic and preventive measures that might well have been derived from research involving risk that, while minor, would be considered more than minimal" (National Commission, 1977). In effect, given the potential benefit to others, the National Commission thought that it was reasonable to allow a parent to permit a child to participate in nonbeneficial research that presented more than a minimal risk. Nevertheless, the National Commission was unwilling to extend this parental authority beyond what was called a "minor increase" over minimal risk.

Paul Ramsey was a prominent critic of the National Commission's decision to allow a parent to enroll a child in nonbeneficial research that presented even a minor increase over minimal risk. According to Ramsey, for a parent to allow a child to undergo any risk for the sake of another person was "a violation of the nature and meaning of the responsibilities of parenthood" (Ramsey, 1970). For a parent to permit such non-beneficial research, "a need or interest on the part of the child-subjects must be discovered if substituted consent has moral warrant. Without that, or without sufficiently competent supplementary consent on the part of the subject accepting the risk, the responsibility of parenthood would be flawed or deflected from its primary role" (Ramsey, 1978). Ramsey later picks up on the suggestion of William Bartholome that participation in research can be "an opportunity for moral growth" (Ramsey, 1978). Thus, a parent may choose to permit a child to participate in non-beneficial research yet remain faithful to the responsibility of parenthood out of a concern for a child's "moral education" (Bartholome, 1977).

The National Commission, in the context of discussing the justification for allowing a child to participate in nontherapeutic research, makes little of the importance of the child's assent apart from the more general requirement for obtaining a child's assent or a parent's permission. Absent the child's assent, the parent would likely be judged as having overstepped the appropriate limits of parental authority. In addition, the stipulation that the research experience be commensurate with a child's actual or routine experience was meant not to increase the risk that the child may justifiably be exposed but to assist children who can assent to make knowledgeable decisions. This suggests that allowable risks are those that the child-subject would judge to be no more than a "minor increase over minimal risk."

The federal regulations, based on the National Commission's report, require both parental permission and child assent except under some clearly defined limits. Assent is defined as the child's "affirmative agreement to participate in research" (45 CFR 46.402(b)). Parental permission and child assent thus function in the pediatric setting as the practical application of the principle of respect for persons, a principle that, in research with competent adult subjects, establishes the requirement for voluntary and informed consent. In the context of research with adults, the requirement for voluntary and informed consent may overprotect certain classes of human subjects, such as those who are unable to provide informed consent yet who may benefit from a research intervention. In the context of research with pediatric subjects, the requirement for assent does not run the risk of overprotection in the therapeutic context as the child's assent may be waived. However, the regulations assume that parental permission (with or without a child's assent) is an insufficient protection against inappropriate research risks. Even when participation in research may directly benefit the child, the IRB is given the responsibility to restrict the available choices to only those research projects that present risks and benefits commensurate with the child's nonresearch alternatives. Finally, nonbeneficial research is restricted to projects presenting no more than minimal risk unless the research may result in important information pertinent to a child's disease or condition, effectively restricting any research involving greater than minimal risk to sick or afflicted children.

Rather than serving as a moral benefit to the child, can a child's assent function as a self-protection mechanism and allow the relaxation of the minimal risk restrictions in pediatric research? It is difficult to arrive at an answer to this question given the absence of agreement on what "assent means." Box 5-1 provides various meanings of the word "assent."

> **BOX 5-1 Definitions of "Assent"**
>
> **Definition from the *Code of Federal Regulations***
>
> "Assent . . . means a child's affirmative agreement to participate in research. Mere failure to object should not, absent affirmative agreement, be construed as assent."
>
> 45 CFR 46.402(b)
>
> **Comment:** As opposed to the extensive guidance on the general requirements for informed consent found in 45 CFR 46.116, there is little discussion of the meaning of assent apart from the brief definition found in Section 46.402(b).
>
> **Definition from the National Commission**
>
> Know that procedures will be performed.
> Choose freely to undergo those procedures.
> Communicate this choice unambiguously.
> Be aware of the option to withdraw.
>
> National Commission, as quoted in Bartholome (1996, p. 356)
>
> **Comment:** This set of recommendations was never incorporated into federal regulations. One of the issues in the discussion of a child's ability to assent or consent to research participation is the developing capacity of the child to "reason" about participation in research. An emphasis on the ability to reason suggests that a child may not consent to research participation until the age of 9 (Leiken, 1993; Weithorn and Campbell, 1982), or when a child is mature enough, for example, to be a "babysitter" (Koren et al., 1993). Note that the above elements of assent as initially discussed by the National Commission do not imply or depend upon a child's ability to reason about the purpose of the research, nor to consider the various risks and benefits of research participation.
>
> **Definition from Bartholome**
>
> Help the child achieve a developmentally appropriate awareness of his/her condition; disclose the nature of the proposed intervention and child's likely experience; assess the child's understanding and any (coercive) factors influencing the child; and solicit the child's unwillingness to accept the proposed intervention.
>
> Bartholome (1996, pp. 360–361)
Continued

> **BOX 5-1** *Continued*
>
> **Comment:** Note that nothing in these four elements of assent requires a sophisticated ability to reason or a sophisticated understanding of the risks and benefits of participation in the research or of the alternatives to participation. As Bartholome points out, the only right that is assumed by the concept of assent is the right to say "no." If a child is capable of reasoning about research participation based on a knowledge of risks and benefits, Bartholome prefers to use the term "consent" (apart from its legal use) to distinguish this level of understanding from "assent."

LEGAL AND REGULATORY CONSIDERATIONS FOR THE CONDUCT OF CLINICAL TRIALS WITH PEDIATRIC POPULATIONS

Presented by Michael Labson, J.D.
Covington & Burling,
Washington, D.C.

In general, the legal system is supportive of research with pediatric populations and provides a great deal of flexibility for such research to be conducted. Nonetheless, the legal system influences research with pediatric populations in two ways: first, by establishing regulatory protections and controls and, second, by providing incentives and requirements to conduct research.

The same general protections that exist for the protection of all human subjects exist for pediatric research subjects, the hallmarks of which are informed consent and IRB review. There are special considerations for informed consent, related to whether to require parental consent, the assent of the child, or both. There are added protections due to the special vulnerability of pediatric patients and special protections for certain subpopulations, like children who are under the care of the state.

Sources for these requirements are the federal policy (45 CFR 46), FDA regulations, some state law, the tort system and the courts, and other nonlegal or extralegal sources, such as professional guidelines.

Subpart D of 45 CFR 46 applies to all DHHS-funded research or research conducted by signatories to the so-called Common Rule. Research is reviewed according to its place under one of four categories: (1) not greater than minimal risk, (2) greater than minimal risk but prospect of direct benefit to the individual subjects, (3) greater than minimal risk and no prospect of direct benefit, but likely to yield generalizable knowledge, and (4) "other."

The first category, research of not greater than minimal risk, requires the assent of the child, when the child is capable. The regulations do not define what a child is but, rather, defer to state law to dictate the age of majority. The determination of capability to assent is determined by criteria established by the local IRB; thus, there is a lot of flexibility. Parental permission for a child's participation in research is also required to be given by one parent or by a legal guardian.

For the second category, greater than minimal risk but prospect of direct benefit, the child's assent (where capable) and parental consent are required, as is IRB review. In addition, the risk must be justified by the anticipated benefit to the subject.

For the third category, no direct benefit but likely to yield generalizable knowledge, the same basic requirements for the previous categories apply but consent or permission of one parent is not sufficient. If there are two parents, the permission of both needs to be obtained. There are added requirements that there be only a minor increase over minimal risk and that the research presents experiences reasonably commensurate with the subject's actual medical experience. The research also must be likely to yield generalizable knowledge of vital importance for the subject's disease or condition.

For research that does not fit into the first three categories, assent of the child, when capable, is required, as is the consent of both parents or legal guardian. In addition, a special requirement holds: a public determination by DHHS that requires expert consultation and public comment to determine that the research presents a reasonable opportunity to further the understanding, prevention, or alleviation of a serious problem that affects children, and that the research will be conducted in accordance with sound ethical principles. As these federal rules illustrate, broad standards exist, but the legal system does not impose specific constraints on research. That task is undertaken by IRBs.

These federal regulations do not preempt state laws. Some states have special requirements that address research with pediatric populations. California's laws might be the broadest, basically prohibiting the use of experimental drugs unless it is related to the health of a subject or obtaining information about the subject's condition. Michigan has a prohibition against nontherapeutic research involving neonates, fetuses, or embryos if it jeopardizes life or health. Illinois has a restriction on the use of purely experimental drugs for minors who are under the care of the state unless use of such a drug is the best chance to save the child's life or treat a serious disease.

The tort system operates against this background. The primary legal theories that are relevant are nonconsensual trespass on the body (battery), and negligence, which can apply even with appropriate informed consent if the responsible researchers or entities are deemed to be exposing their patients to undue risk in violation of the duty to care that they owe to their patients. There is little case law in this area.

In addition to these regulatory protections and controls on pediatric research, the law creates incentives and requirements to perform research. FDAMA (PL 105–115) contains provisions that establish economic incentives for conducting studies with pediatric populations with drugs for which exclusivity or patent protection is available under the Drug Price Competition and Patent Term Restoration Act (PL 98-417) and the Orphan Drug Act (PL 97-414). These provisions extend by 6 months any existing exclusivity or patent protection for a drug for which FDA has requested studies with a pediatric population and the manufacturer has conducted such studies in accordance with the requirements of FDAMA. This exclusivity will be particularly important in encouraging companies to study formulations and dosing for study patients.

Manufacturers are eligible for exclusivity under FDAMA when they submit the results of a study to FDA in response to FDA's written request for such a study. The study results are not required to provide useful information on use by pediatric patients (e.g., the results may be inconclusive), and the sponsor is not required to obtain approval for the addition of the information gained in the study to the drug's label.

In addition to the incentives of FDAMA for studies with pediatric populations, FDA has promulgated a regulation mandating that manufacturers conduct studies of certain products with pediatric populations. The rule establishes a presumption that all new drugs and biologics will be studied in pediatric patients, but allows manufacturers to obtain a waiver of the requirement if the product does not represent a meaningful therapeutic benefit over existing treatments for pediatric patients and is not likely to be used by a substantial number of pediatric patients. The rule also provides that FDA will require studies of already marketed drugs under "compelling circumstances."

As described in FDA's earlier 1994 rule on labeling for pediatric patient use, the gathering of adequate data to establish safety and effectiveness for pediatric populations may not require controlled clinical trials with pediatric patients. When the course of the disease and the product's effects are similar in adults and pediatric patients, FDA may conclude that safety and effectiveness for pediatric patients can be supported by effectiveness data for adults together with additional data, such as dosing, pharmacokinetic, and safety data for pediatric patients. The new rule does not necessarily require separate studies with pediatric patients. In appropriate cases, adequate data may be gathered by including pediatric patients as well as adults in the original studies conducted on the product.

The mandatory study rule requires studies with pediatric populations for new and marketed drugs and biologics, effective April 1, 1999, with data by December 2000, unless a deferral is granted. Studies must cover each age group for which the studies would be likely to produce a meaningful therapeutic benefit or for which the product is used by a substantial number of pediatric patients. This includes the stipulation that companies may be required to develop a new formulation. The rule also requires that sponsors submit postmarketing reports.

One of the controversial legal issues presented by the mandatory rule is whether FDA has the authority to require studies when a sponsor is not coming forward and proposing the studies or when a sponsor is not proposing the placement of indications on its labeling for pediatric patients. No legal challenge has been brought to the rule. However, it is possible that in individual cases a company might challenge FDA's authority to require pediatric studies.

Although it is too early to draw definitive conclusions about FDA's current research initiative for pediatric populations, it holds great promise to improve drug labeling for pediatric patients. The incentives in FDAMA in particular provide a powerful engine to drive research initiatives for pediatric populations and place them on a par with competing research demands.

INTERNATIONAL DEVELOPMENT OF DRUGS FOR PEDIATRIC PATIENTS: AN INDUSTRY PERSPECTIVE

Stephen P. Spielberg, M.D., Ph.D.
*Vice President, Pediatric Drug Development,
Janssen Research Foundation*

The International Conference on Harmonization (ICH) is a tripartite effort to harmonize the process of drug development in the United States, Europe, and Japan. There is also representation from Canada and from European countries that are not members of the European Union. In terms of regulations for pediatric populations, its goal is the international availability of standardized, validated formulations for use by pediatric populations and of drug evaluation standards that permit the use and the regulatory acceptability of similar protocols internationally.

An example of why this is needed is provided by the differences between Canada and the United States on two types of sweeteners. On the basis of analyses with identical data, saccharin was approved for use in the United States and cyclamates were banned, but in Canada saccharin was banned and cyclamates were approved. This means that if a U.S. product is sweetened with saccharin, it cannot be sold in Canada.

Another pressing concern is that many of the children live in places where refrigeration is not available. Thus, if medicines are stable only under refrigerated conditions, those medicines are not going to be usable by most of the children in the world.

A third concern had to do with the generalizability of the data derived from clinical trials conducted in one country in terms of application in other countries. There is a need for pediatric investigators to have the ability to work together, on an international scale, by using the same validated formulations, with defined bioavailability and stability, and by studying medications under similar protocols. Application of pediatric pharmaceuticals on a global scale necessitates the acceptability of formulations and requires that the data generated from such international trials for labeling purposes be internationally accepted.

As one of its first tasks, the ICH pediatric working group reviewed current international regulatory documents on development of drugs for children to identify areas of consensus and disagreement and to try to negotiate a document that would be acceptable to all participants.

The working group was able to reach consensus, signing off on a "Step 2" document (ICH E-11: Investigation of Medicinal Products in the Pediatric Population) in October 1999. The document will now go through a 6-month comment period in the United States, the European Union, and Japan; on the basis of input, a final document to be adopted by ICH will then be prepared. The general principles set forth in the document reaffirm that safe and effective pharmacotherapy in children requires studies with children; indeed, not to do such studies places children at greater risk from therapeutic misadventures with nonvalidated treatments. The ethical imperative to obtain needed information in clinical studies must be balanced against the ethical imperative to protect each child in such studies.

The document discusses several critical issues in development of drugs for pediatric populations: timing of initiation of studies with pediatric populations in the process of overall drug development; development of pediatric formulations, types of studies (pharmacokinetic, pharmacokinetic-pharmacodynamic, efficacy, safety), and the age categories of the patients to be studied. In addition, there is a section on special ethical considerations in studies with pediatric populations, including the role and composition of IRBs, recruitment of subjects, parental consent (permission) and assent of the child, and approaches to minimizing risk and distress and maximizing the benefit for children in studies. In the latter context, there is discussion about the nature of investigative sites where children should be studied, the training and expertise of personnel, and assurance that being a patient in a clinical study is made as positive an experience for the child as possible.

Regulatory and legislative initiatives in the United States have had a major impact on development of drugs for pediatric populations. The 1997 FDAMA included provisions for an incentive to industry in the form of a 6-month extension of marketing exclusivity for performance of pediatric studies. Since its inception, more than 100 drugs not previously labeled for use by children are now being evaluated. The 1998 FDA Pediatric Rule contains additional provisions to ensure that medicines that are important for children and that will be used by pediatricians will have appropriate information on their safe and effective use. With the increase in investigative activity that has occurred, it is the hope that ICH E-11 can provide a framework for international cooperation on clinical investigations with pediatric populations for the benefit of all the world's children.

PANEL DISCUSSION

Many new agents are in the pharmaceutical development pipeline. Because of changes in federal regulations and in response to incentives, it is likely that many of these agents will be studied for use in children. This changing environment, although promising, raises issues and concerns in several areas.

The Need for Trained Research Personnel

A skilled cadre of pediatric clinical pharmacologists will be required to achieve the goals established by new regulatory policies. With the new FDA rule (Pediatric Rule), every drug coming through the pipeline will require appropriate evaluation for use by pediatric populations. That is going to necessitate a new generation of pediatric clinical pharmacologists. Academic health centers will have to provide incentives and rewards for those investigators who conduct research with pediatric populations in multicenter studies.

Improved Study Design

Single-dose studies with children deserve additional considerations from both ethical and scientific perspectives. They raise concerns about the likelihood of benefit to a particular child or patient population, yet in some cases they might be the only way to obtain valuable clinical data. The need for and value of phase I trials with single-dose studies remain controversial because of the risk that a clinical trial could be started with the wrong dose. The drug then could erroneously be deemed ineffective or the entire trial may need to be repeated with a larger cohort of patients with a new dose.

Errors made in past studies with pediatric populations have largely resulted from the fact that trials were started before adequate pharmacokinetic studies had been conducted. Such errors are hazardous and expose more children to risk than do concentrated, smaller studies. Although study size should always be kept to a minimum, statistics, biochemistry, and pharmacology should dictate study size.

Obtaining the needed enrollment in pediatric studies can be daunting, as the pool of available patients can be small. Good models are provided by the Pediatric Oncology Group and the National Institute of Child Health and Human Development neonatal network, which provides linkages among neonatologists to conduct studies with larger numbers of patients.

In 1991 the Institute of Medicine Forum on Drug Development recommended that National Institutes of Health establish a means of solving the problem of the historic lack of information about drug development for infants and children. As a consequence, the National Institute of Child Health and Human Development established a pediatric pharmacology research network. The network encompasses many of the leading pediatric clinical pharmacologists at universities and children's hospitals in the United States. Thus, it can draw on the data from the more than 200,000 inpatient and 2 million pediatric outpatient visits each year.

Role of Insurance and Managed Care Organizations

In some areas of the United States, health insurance providers report spending more on pharmaceutical coverage than inpatient hospital services. In trying to address the rapidly growing cost of prescription pharmaceuticals, some insurers and managed care organizations have begun to develop more restrictive formularies, basically applying tiered payments to offer incentives for the purchase of preferred pharmaceuticals. Thus, insurers have an interest in encouraging safe and efficient clinical testing of drugs for use by the pediatric population. One way of building on the incentives already being supplied through FDAMA would be to encourage the use of pharmaceuticals that have received guidance and labeling instructions for administration to pediatric patients. Some have suggested that third party payers should perhaps stop paying for either off-label or innovative interventions unless they are used as part of a well designed, controlled, and adequate study. Other providers have established policies that do not deny payment to any patient participating in any phase I through IV clinical trials. In New Jersey, for example, insurance and managed care organizations have agreed not to exclude patients from coverage for health care needed because of participation in certain phases of clinical trials. Standard contracts often exclude patients from coverage when they participate in clinical trials.

Legal Concerns

Legal questions remain: What will the effect of the mandatory study rule be, particularly for marketed products? Will the FDAMA incentive be renewed after its initial impact is evaluated?

International Issues

Although the ethics of research with children will always differ among cultures and nations, the fundamental principles of how such research should be done can be developed. In any event, ethical issues should be openly discussed. The World Medical Association and the American Medical Association have established a task force to receive and review input on the Helsinki Declaration in an effort to achieve some standardization of basic ethical principles for research with humans.

6

Concluding Remarks

Presented by Murray M. Lumpkin, M.D.
*Deputy Center Director,
Center for Drug Evaluation and Research,
U.S. Food and Drug Administration*

For too long, pediatricians have all too often been prescribing medications to their patients on the basis of insufficient clinical research data. In addition, there has been a lack of standardized pediatric formulations for many drugs; insufficient data to support dosing, efficacy, and precaution statements; and lingering and persistent concerns about the disclaimers put in labeling and promotion, despite the widespread use of these products for pediatric patients. When a child is given a prescription drug under these circumstances, he or she is essentially being used as a nonconsenting participant in an "*N*-of-one" trial.

This past record is shameful. However, the discussion at this workshop has demonstrated a sense that the government and the pharmaceutical industry have a shared interest and mutual desire to use newly acquired legislative and regulatory tools to improve this record.

Even with this shared interest, however, serious issues must be resolved if real progress is to be made. Legal and ethical concerns pertaining to institutional review board review and informed consent must be resolved. Careful attention must be paid to recruitment incentives, clinical trial designs, the use of placebos, and the sufficiency of the data required for use of a drug by adults before children are involved.

The workshop has raised concerns about whether sufficient numbers of pediatric patients and sufficient numbers of qualified clinical researchers can be recruited to carry out the ambitious studies that workshop participants agreed were desirable. Although participants expressed optimism that new laboratory methodologies have been developed to make drug testing more applicable to children, they also expressed concern about the lack of appropriate formulations and commercial incentives for the development of some drugs that are of high import to the pediatric population but not covered by the new legislative incentives.

It is very important that the extension of marketing exclusivity granted under the Food and Drug Administration Modernization Act (FDAMA) to sponsors of certain pediatric drugs be carefully evaluated to make sure that it is being used appropriately for a societal good. It has been a tool used by the U.S. Congress in the past to promote the development of orphan and generic drugs. Now, for the third time, the Congress is using this tool to encourage the development of drugs for use in infants and children.

This financial incentive carries with it a serious scientific responsibility to implement it effectively in the public interest. It is likely to result in changes in attitudes about the feasibility of studies with children and, as a result, a larger infrastructure for studying the effects of drugs in children. Health care professionals should all be held accountable for how well this authority is used. It is hoped that this will result in better labeling of drugs for use by the pediatric population, more appropriate formulations, better dosing guidelines for more age ranges, and better information about efficacy and toxicity of drugs in children.

The U.S. Food and Drug Administration (FDA) is required to submit a report to the Congress by January 1, 2001, on how well this FDAMA provision has worked to improve information regarding pediatric uses of drugs. The Congress will want to know whether the exclusivity tool was used well and whether the children of the United States have benefited. If the result does not meet expectations, it could be said that children were exploited for the financial gain of a few corporations. However, failure is not expected or the many challenges that will need to be met. The following four challenges will be the most difficult to address:

- Some good metrics must be developed to determine whether the goals of the new incentive programs have been met.
- If heavy reliance on extrapolation of data from adult populations is used to establish efficacy in children, there must be a way of evaluating, over the long term, whether this was a valid surrogate.
- Longer-term follow-up studies must be developed, financed, and conducted to assess the effect of drugs on unique pediatric safety issues such as children's growth and their neuronal, psychosocial, and endocrinologic maturation.
- If it is concluded that this incentive program is effective in spurring the development and appropriate use of drugs in the pediatric population and that it is worth the overall cost to society, the question of whether it should be applied to other populations (such as pregnant women, elderly people, or members of minority groups) and, if so, whether doing so will it be at the expense of maintaining the program for children, will need to be addressed.

References

Agertoft, L., and S. Pedersen. 1994. Effects of long term treatment with an inhaled corticosteroid on growth and pulmonary function in asthmatic children. *Respiratory Medicine* 88:373–381.

American Academy of Pediatrics, Committee on Drugs. 1977. Guidelines for the ethical conduct of studies to evaluate drugs in pediatric populations. *Pediatrics* 60:91–101.

American Academy of Pediatrics, Committee on Drugs. 1995. Guidelines for the ethical conduct of studies to evaluate drugs in pediatric populations (RE9503). *Pediatrics* 95(2):286–294.

Andersson, K. E., A. Bertler, and G. Wettrell. 1975. Post-mortem distribution and tissue concentrations of digoxin in infants and adults. *Acta Paediatrica Scandinavica* 64(3):497–504.

Aranda, J. V., J. M. Collinge, R. Zinman, and G. Watters. 1979. Maturation of caffeine elimination in infancy. *Archives of Disease in Children* 54:946–949.

Bajpai, M., L. K. Roskos, D. D. Shen, and R. H. Levy. 1996. Roles of cytochrome P4502C9 and cytochrome P4502C19 in the stereoselective metabolism of phenytoin to its major metabolite. *Drug Metabolism and Disposition* 24:1401–1403.

Bartholome, W. G. 1977. The ethics of non-therapeutic clinical research on children. In *Appendix to Report and Recommendations: Research Involving Children*. The National Commission for the Protection of Human Subjects of Biomedical and Behavioral Research. DHEW Publication No. (OS) 77-0005:3–17.

Bartholome, W. G. 1996. Ethical issues in pediatric research. In *The Ethics of Research Involving Human Subjects*. Edited by Harold Y. Vanderpool. Frederick, Md.: University Publishing Group. 356, 360–361.

Bourgeois, B. F. D., and W. E. Dodson. 1983. Phenytoin elimination in newborns. *Neurology* 33:173–178.

Brown, R. D., G. L. Kearns, and J. T. Wilson. 1993. Integrated pharmacokinetic (PKN)/pharmacodynamic (PDN) model for acetaminophen and ibuprofen antipyresis in children. *Clinical Pharmacology and Therapeutics* 53.

Brown, R. D., G. L. Kearns, and J. T. Wilson. 1998. Integrated pharmacokinetic-pharmacodynamic model for acetaminophen, ibuprofen, and placebo antipyresis in children. *Journal of Pharmacokinetics and Biopharmacology* 25:559.

Burtin, P., E. Jacqz-Aigrain, P. Girard, R. Lenclen, J. F. Magny, P. Betremieux, C. Tehiry, L. Desplanques, and P. Mussat. 1994. Population pharmacokinetics of midazolam in neonates. *Clinical Pharmacology and Therapeutics* 56:615–625.

Busse, W., S. P. Banks-Schlegel, and G. L. Larsen. 1995. Childhood versus adult-onset asthma. *American Journal of Respiratory Critical Care Medicine* 151:1635–1639.

Cazenave, C., G. Pons, E. Rey, J. M. Treluyer, T. Cresteil, G. Thiroux, P. D'Athis, and G. Olive. 1994. Biotransformation of caffeine in human liver microsomes from fetuses, neonates, infants and adults. *British Journal of Clinical Pharmacology* 37:405–412.

Chiba, K., T. Ishizaki, H. Miura, and K. Minigawa. 1980. Michaelis-Menten pharmacokinetics of diphenylhydantoin and application in the pediatric age patient. *Journal of Pediatrics* 96:479–484.

Craig, W. A. and D. Andes. 1996. Pharmacokinetics and pharmacodynamics of antibiotics in otitis media. *Pediatric Infectious Disease Journal* 15(3):255–259.

Cresteil, T. 1998. Onset of xenobiotic metabolism in children: Toxicological implications. *Food Additives and Contaminates* 15(Suppl.):45–51.

Cresteil, T. 1999. The development of metabolic mechanisms for xenobiotics. *Nestle Nutrition Workshop Series,* Vol. 44.

Cresteil, T., P. Beaune, P. Kremers, J. P. Flinois, and J. P. Leroux. 1982. Drug-metabolizing enzymes in human fetal liver: Partial resolution of multiple cytochromes P-450. *Pediatric Pharmacology* 2:199–207.

Cresteil, T., P. Beaune, P. Kremers, C. Celier, F. P. Guengerich, and J. P. Leroux. 1985. Immunoquantification of epoxide hydrolase and cytochrome P-450 isozymes in fetal and adult human liver microsomes. *European Journal of Biochemistry* 151:345–350.

Cumming, R. G., P. Mitchell, and S. R. Leeder. 1997. Use of inhaled corticosteroids and the risk of cataracts. *New England Journal of Medicine* 337:8–14.

de Wildt, S. N., G. L. Kearns, J. S. Leeder, and J. N. van den Anker. 1999a. Glucuronidation in humans: Pharmacogenetic and developmental aspects. *Clinical Pharmacokinetics* 36:439–452.

de Wildt, S. N., G. L. Kearns, J. S. Leeder, and J. N. van den Anker. 1999b. Cytochrome P450 3A: Ontogeny and drug disposition. *Clinical Pharmacokinetics* 37(6):485–505.

DHHS (U.S. Department of Health and Human Services). 1983. Federal Policy for the Protection of Human Subjects: Additional Protections for Children Involved as Subjects in Research. *Federal Register* 48:9818. (codified at 45 CFR §46.404–406).

DHHS. 1991a. Federal Policy for the Protection of Human Subjects: Basic Policy for the Protection of Human Research Subjects. *Federal Register* 56:28003. (codified at 45 CFR §46A).

DHHS. 1991b. Federal Policy for the Protection of Human Subjects: Additional Protections for Children Involved as Subjects in Research (Technical Amendment). *Federal Register* 56:28032. (codified at 45 CFR §46.404–406).

DuBuske, L. M., J. Grossman, and L. M. Dube. 1997. Randomized trial in patients with moderate asthma: Effect of reduced dosing frequency and amounts on pulmonary function and asthma symptoms. *American Journal of Managed Care* 3:633–640.

Ellenberg, S. S., N. Geller, R. Simon, and S. Yusuf (eds). 1993. Proceedings of "Practical Issues in Data Monitoring of Clinical Trials." *Statistics in Medicine* 12:415–616.

FDA (U.S. Food and Drug Administration). 1992. New drug antibiotic and biological drug product regulations: Accelerated approval. Proposed Rule 57 *Federal Register*.

FDA. 1996. *Guidance for Industry: E6 Good Clinical Practice: Consolidated Guidance*. Bethesda, Md.: Center for Drug Evaluation and Research and Center for Biologics Evaluation and Research. April 1996.

FDA. 1997a. Food and Drug Administration Modernization Act of 1997. Section III. The pediatric exclusivity provision.

FDA. 1997b. Good clinical practice: Consolidated guidance (FDA guidance document). *Federal Register* 62:25691–25709.

FDA. 1998a. Pulmonary and Allergy and Endocrinology Advisory Committees Meeting. Bethesda, Md.: U.S. Food and Drug Administration. July 30–31, 1998.

FDA. 1998b. *Draft Guidance: General Considerations for Pediatric Pharmacokinetic Studies for Drugs and Biological Products*. Bethesda, Md.: U.S. Food and Drug Administration. November 10, 1998.

FDA. 1998c. *Guidance for Industry: General Considerations for Pediatric Pharmacokinetic Studies for Drugs and Biological Products*. Bethesda, Md.: Center for Drug Evaluation and Research and Center for Biologics Evaluation and Research. November, 1998.

FDA. 1998d. Statistical principles for clinical trials (FDA guidance document). *Federal Register* 63: 49583–49598.

FDA. 1998e. Regulations requiring manufacturers to assess the safety and effectiveness of new drugs and biological products in pediatric patients. 63 *Federal Register* 66632–66672. (codified at 21CFR Parts 201, 312, 314 and 601).

FDA. 1999. *Guidance for Industry: Population Pharmacokinetics*. Bethesda, Md.: Center for Drug Evaluation and Research and Center for Biologics Evaluation and Research. February 1999.

Fleming, T. R. and D. L. DeMets. 1993. Monitoring of clinical trials: Issues and recommendations. *Controlled Clinical Trials* 14(3):183–197.

Forrest, A., D. E. Nix, C. H. Ballow, T. F. Goss, M. C. Birmingham, and J. J. Schentag. 1993. Pharmacodynamics of intravenous ciprofloxacin in seriously ill patients. *Antimicrobial Agents and Chemotherapy* 37:1073–1081.

Freedman, B. 1987. Equipoise and the ethics of clinical research. *New England Journal of Medicine* 317(3):141–145.

Fritz, S., W. Lindner, I. Roots, B. M. Frey, and A. Küpfer. 1987. Stereochemistry of aromatic phenytoin hydroxylation in various drug hydroxylation phenotypes in humans. *Journal of Pharmacology and Experimental Therapies* 241:615–622.

Garbe, E., J. LeLorier, J.F. Boivin, and S. Suissa. 1997. Inhaled and nasal glucocorticoids and the risks of ocular hypertension or open-angle glaucoma. *Journal of the American Medical Association* 277:722–727.

Garbe, E., S. Suissa, and J. LeLorier. 1998. Association of inhaled corticosteroid use with cataract extraction in elderly patients. *Journal of the American Medical Association* 280:539–543.

Gorodischer, R., W. J. Jusko, and S. J. Yaffe. 1976. Tissue and erythrocyte distribution of digoxin in infants. *Clinical Pharmacology and Therapeutics* 19(3):256–264.

Gotschall, R. R., J. S. Leeder, S. M. Abdel-Rahman, M. McCubbin, M. D. Reed, H. C. Farrar, and G. L. Kearns. 1999a. CYP1A2 activity in cystic fibrosis: Lack of concordance with caffeine plasma clearance. *Pediatric Pulmonology* (Suppl. 19):210.

Gotschall, R. R., K. Marcucci, J. S. Leeder, and G. L. Kearns. 1999b. Cisapride biotransformation: Not all CYP3As are created equal. *Clinical Pharmacology and Therapeutics* 65:127.

Green, S. J., T. R. Fleming, and J. R. O'Fallon. 1987. Policies for study monitoring and interim reporting of results. *Journal of Clinical Oncology* 5(9):1477–1484.

Haahtela, T., M. Jarvinen, T. Kava, K. Kiviranta, S. Koskinen, K. Lehtonen, K. Nikander, T. Persson, O. Selroos, and A. Sovijarvi. 1994. Effects of reducing or discontinuing inhaled budesonide in patients with mild asthma. *New England Journal of Medicine* 331:700–705.

Hakkola, J., M. Pasanen, R. Purkunen, S. Saarikoski, O. Pelkonen, J. Maenpaa, A. Rane, and H. Raunio. 1994. Expression of xenobiotic-metabolizing cytochrome P450 forms in human adult and fetal liver. *Biochemical Pharmacology* 48:59–64.

Hamilton, A., I. Faiferman, P. Stober, R. M. Watson, and P. M. O'Byrne. 1998. Pranlukast, a cysteinyl leukotriene receptor antagonist, attenuates allergen-induced early and late phase bronchoconstriction and airway hyperresponsiveness in asthmatic subjects. *Journal of Allergy and Clinical Immunology* 102:177–183.

Holgate, S. T., P. Bradding, and A. P. Sampson. 1996. Leukotriene antagonists and synthesis inhibitors: New directions in asthma therapy. *Journal of Allergy and Clinical Immunology* 98:1–13.

ICH E-11: Investigation of Medicinal Products in the Pediatric Population. October 1999.

In, K. H., K. Asano, D. Beier, J. Grobholz, P. W. Finn, E. K. Silverman, E. S. Silverman, T. Collins, A. R. Fischer, T. P. Keith, K. Serino, S. W. Kim, G. T. De Sanctis, C. Yandava, A. Pillari, P. Rubin, J. Kemp, E. Israel, W. Busse, D. Ledford, J. J. Murray, A. Segal, D. Tinkleman, and J. M. Drazen. 1997. Naturally occurring mutations in the human 5-lipoxygenase gene promoter that modify transcription factor binding and reporter gene transcription. *Journal of Clinical Investigation* 99(5):1130–1137.

Israel, E., J. Cohn, L. Dube, and J. M. Drazen. 1996. Effect of treatment with zileuton, a 5-lipoxygenase inhibitor, in patients with asthma. A randomized controlled trial. Zileuton Clinical Trial Group. *Journal of the American Medical Association* 275:931–936.

Jacqz-Aigrain, E., C. Funck-Brentano, and T. Cresteil. 1993. CYP2D6 and CYP3A-dependent metabolism of dextromethorphan in humans: Fetal and adult studies. *Pharmacogenetics* 3:197–204.

Kashuba, A. D. M., A. N. Nafziger, and G. L. Kearns. 1998. Effect of fluvoxamine therapy on the activities of CYP1A2, CYP2D6 and CYP3A as determined by phenotyping. *Clinical Pharmacology and Therapeutics* 64:257–268.

Kearns, G. L. 1998. Pharmacokinetics in infants and children. *Inflammatory Bowel Diseases* 4(2):104–107.

Kearns, G. L., D. J. Murry, C. Oermann, A. Gaedigh, M. Sockrider, D. K. Seilheimer, and J. S. Leeder. 1999. Ibuprofen pharmacokinetics in cystic fibrosis: Association with CYP2C9 genotype. *Pediatric Pulmonology* (Suppl. 19):208.

Kemp, J.P., R. J. Dockhorn, G. G. Shapiro, H. H. Nguyen, T. F. Reiss, B.C. Seidenberg, and B. Knorr. 1998. Montelukast once daily inhibits exercise-induced bronchoconstriction in 6- to 14-year-old children with asthma. *Journal of Pediatrics* 133:424–428.

Kerr, B. M., K. E. Thummel, C. J. Wurden, S. M. Klein, D. L. Kroetz, F. J. Gonzalez, and R. H. Levy. 1994. Human liver carbamazepine metabolism. Role of CYP3A4 and CYP2C8 in 10,11-epoxide formation. *Biochemistry and Pharmacology* 47:1969–1979.

Kinirons, M. T., D. O'Shea, R. B. Kim, J. D. Groopman, K. E. Thummel, A. J. J. Wood, and G. R. Wilkinson. 1999. Failure of erythromycin breath test to correlate with midazolam clearance as a probe of cytochrome P4503A. *Clinical Pharmacology and Therapeutics* 66:224–231.

Knorr, B., J. Matz, and J. A. Bernstein. 1998. Montelukast for chronic asthma in 6- to 14-year-old children: A randomized, double-blind trial. Pediatric Montelukast Study Group. *Journal of the American Medical Association* 279:1181–1186.

Kolars, J. C., K. C. Lown, P. Schmiedlin-Ren, M. Ghosh, C. Fang, S. A. Wrighton, R. M. Merion, and P. B. Watkins. 1994. CYP3A gene expression in human gut epithelium. *Pharmacogenetics* 4:247–259.

Komori, M., K. Nishio, M. Kitada, K. Shiramatsu, K. Muroya, M. Soma, K. Nagashima, and T. Kamataki. 1990. Fetus-specific expression of a form of cytochrome P-450 in human livers. *Biochemistry* 29:4430–4433.

Koren, G., D.B. Carmeli, Y.S. Carmeli, and R. Haslam. 1993. Maturity of children to consent to medical research: The babysitter test. *Journal of Medical Ethics* 19(3):142–147.

Korinthenberg, R., C. Haug, and D. Hannak. 1994. The metabolization of carbamazepine to CBZ-10,11-epoxide in children from the newborn age to adolescence. *Neuropediatrics* 25:214–216.

Kraus, D. M., J. H. Fischer, S. J. Reitz, S. A. Kecskes, T. F. Yeh, K. M. McCulloch, E. C. Tung, and M. J. Cwik. 1993. Alterations in theophylline metabolism during the first year of life. *Clinical Pharmacology and Therapeutics* 54:351–359.

Kroetz, D. L., B. M. Kerr, and L. V. McFarland. 1993. Measurement of in-vivo microsomal epoxide hydrolase activity in white subjects. *Clinical Pharmacology and Therapeutics* 53:306–315.

Lacroix, D., M. Sonnier, A. Moncion, G. Cheron, and T. Cresteil. 1997. Expression of CYP3A in the human liver: Evidence that the shift between CYP3A7 and CYP3A4 occurs immediately after birth. *European Journal of Biochemistry* 247: 625–634.

Laitinen, A., A. Altraja, M. Kampe, M. Linden, I. Virtanen, and L. Laitinen. 1997. Tenascin is increased in airway basement membrane of asthmatics and decreased by an inhaled steroid. *American Journal of Respiratory Critical Care Medicine* 156:951–958.

Lambert, G. H., D. A. Schoeller, and A. N. Kotake. 1986. The effect of age, gender and sexual maturation on the caffeine breath test. *Developmental Pharmacology and Therapeutics* 9:375–381.

Lange, P., J. Parner, J. Vestbo, P. Schnohr, and G. Jensen. 1998. A 15-year follow-up study of ventilatory function in adults with asthma. *New England Journal of Medicine* 339:1194–1200.

Le Guennec, J. C., and B. Billon. 1987. Delay in caffeine elimination in breast-fed infants. *Pediatrics* 79:264–268.
Lee, T. H., R. Brattsand, and D. Leung. 1996. Corticosteroid action and resistance in asthma. *American Journal of Respiratory and Critical Care Medicine* 154 (Suppl.):S1–S79.
Leeder, J. S., and G. L. Kearns. 1997. Pharmacogenetics in pediatrics: Implications for practice. *Pediatric Clinics of North America* 44:55–77.
Leff, R. D., L. J. Fischer, and R. J. Roberts. 1986. Phenytoin metabolism in infants following intravenous and oral administration. *Developmental Pharmacology and Therapeutics* 9:217–223.
Leikin, S. 1993. Minors' assent, consent, or dissent to medical research. *IRB: A Review of Human Subjects Research* 15(2):1–7.
Leung, D. Y. M., R. J. Martin, S. J. Szefler, E. R. Sher, S. Ying, A. B. Kay, and Q. Hamid. 1995. Dysregulation of inteleukin-4, interleukin-2, and interferon-g gene expression in steroid-resistant asthma. *Journal of Experimental Medicine* 181:33–40.
Liu, M. C., L. M. Dube, J. Lancaster, and the Zileuton Study Group. 1996. Acute and chronic effects of a 5-lipoxygenase inhibitor in asthma: 6-month randomized multicenter trial. *Journal of Allergy and Clinical Immunology* 98:859–871.
Loughnan, P. M., A. Greenwald, W. W. Purton, J. V. Aranda, G. Watters, and A. H. Neims. 1977. Pharmacokinetic observations of phenytoin disposition in the newborn and young infant. *Archives of Disease in Childhood* 52:302–309.
Mäenpää, J. V. A., O. Pelkonen, T. Cresteil, and A. Rane. 1993. The role of cytochrome P4503A (CYP3A) isoform(s) in oxidative metabolism of testosterone and benzphetamine in adult and fetal liver. *Journal of Steroid Biochemistry and Molecular Biology* 44:61–67.
McLeod, H. L., E. Y. Krynetski, and J. A. Wilimas. 1995. Higher activity of polymorphic thiopruine S-methyltransferase in erythrocytes from neonates compared to adults. *Pharmacogenetics* 5:281–286.
Meinert, C. L. 1998. Clinical trials and treatment effects monitoring (with discussion). *Controlled Clinical Trials* 19:515–543.
Milsap, R. L., and W. J. Jusko. 1994. Pharmacokinetics in the infant. *Environmental Health Perspectives* 102 (Suppl. 11):107–110.
Murry, D. J., W. R. Crom, W. E. Reddick, R. Bhargava, and W. E. Evans. 1995. Liver volume as a determinant of drug clearance in children and adolescents. *Drug Metabolism and Disposition* 23:1110–1116.
Nakamura, H., A. Hasegawa, M. Kimura, S. Yamagata, H. Nakasa, H. Osada, S. Sekiya, S. Ohmori, and M. Kitada. 1999. Comparison of urinary 6ß-hydroxycortisol/cortisol ratio between neonates and their mothers. *British Journal of Clinical Pharmacology* 47:31–34.
Nakamura, H., M. Hirai, S. Ohmori, Y. Ohsone, T. Obonai, K. Sugita, H. Niimi, and M. Kitada. 1998a. Changes in urinary 6ß-hydroxycortisol/cortisol ratio after birth in human neonates. *European Journal of Clinical Pharmacology* 53:343–346.
Nakamura, Y., M. Hoshino, J. Joon Sim, K. Ishii, K. Hosaka, and T. Sakamoto. 1998b. Effect of the leukotriene receptor antagonist pranlukast on cellular infiltration in the bronchial mucosa of patients with asthma. *Thorax* 53:835–841.

Nassif, E. G., M. M. Weinberger, D. Shannon, S. F. Guiang, L. Hendeles, D. Jimenez, and E. Ekwo. 1981. Theophylline disposition in infancy. *Journal of Pediatrics* 98:158–161.

National Commission (National Commission for the Protection of Human Subjects of Biomedical and Behavioral Research). 1977. *Report and Recommendations: Research Involving Children.* DHEW Publication No. 77-0004. 5–7, 126–127, 137.

National Commission. 1979. The Belmont Report: Ethical Principles and Guidelines for the Protection of Human Subjects. *Federal Register Doc.* 79:12065. April 18, 1979. xx.

National Heart, Lung, and Blood Institute. 1995. *Global Strategy for Asthma Management and Prevention.* Workshop Report. Publication No. 95-3659. Bethesda, Md.: National Heart Lung and Blood Institute.

National Heart, Lung, and Blood Institute. 1997. *National Asthma Education and Prevention Program Expert Panel Report II: Guidelines for the Diagnosis and Management of Asthma.* Publication No. 97-4051. Bethesda, Md.: National Heart, Lung, and Blood Institute.

Nelson, H. S., I. L. Bernstein, J. Fink, T. B. Edwards, S. L. Spector, W. W. Storms, and D. P. Tashkin for the Pulmicort Turbuhaler Study Group. 1998. Oral glucocorticosteroid-sparing effect of budesonide administered by Turbuhaler. *Chest* 113:1264–1271.

Nelson, R.M. 1998. Children as research subjects. Pp. 47–66 in *Beyond Consent: Seeking Justice in Research*, J. Kahn, A. Mastroianni, and J. Sugarman, eds. New York: Oxford University Press.

Noonan, M., P. Chervinsky, and W. W. Busse. 1995. Fluticasone propionate reduces oral prednisone use while it improves asthma control and quality of life. *American Journal of Respiratory Critical Care Medicine* 152:1467–1473.

Olivierie, D., A. Chetta, M. Del Donno, et al. 1997. Effect of short-term treatment with low-dose inhaled fluticasone propionate on airway inflammation and remodeling in mild asthma: A placebo-controlled study. *American Journal of Respiratory Critical Care Medicine* 155:1864–1871.

Overbeek, S. E., H. A. M. Kerstjens, J. M. Bogaard, P. G. H. Mulder, D. S. Postma, and the Dutch CNSLD study group. 1996. Is delayed introduction of inhaled corticosteroids harmful in patients with obstructive airways disease (asthma and COPD)? *Chest* 110:35–41.

Pariente-Khayat, A., G. Pons, E. Rey, M. Richard, P. d'Athis, L. Moran, J. Badoual, and G. Olive. 1991. Caffeine acetylator phenotyping during maturation in infants. *Pediatric Research* 29:492–496.

Park-Hah, J. O., B. Klemetsdal, R. Lysaa, K. H. Choi, and J. Aarbakke. 1996. Thiopurine methyltransferase activity in a Korean population sample of children. *Clinical Pharmacology and Therapeutics* 60:68–74.

Payne, K., F. J. Mattheyse, D. Liedenberg, and T. Dawes. 1989. The pharmacokinetics of midazolam in paediatric patients. *European Journal of Clinical Pharmacology* 37:267–272.

Peat, J. 1998. Asthma: A longitudinal perspective. *Journal of Asthma* 35:235–241.

Pedersen, S., and O. R. Hansen. 1995. Budesonide treatment of moderate and severe asthma in children: A dose-response study. *Journal of Allergy and Clinical Immunology* 95:29–33.

Pelkonen, O., E. H. Kaltiala, T. K. I. Larmi, and N. T. Karki. 1973. Comparison of activities of drug-metabolizing enzymes in human fetal and adult livers. *Clinical Pharmacology and Therapeutics* 14:840–846.

Pynnönen, S., M. Sillanpää, H. Frey, and E. Iisalo. 1977. Carbamazepine and its 10,11-epoxide in children and adults with epilepsy. *European Journal of Clinical Pharmacology* 11:129–133.

Ramsey, P. 1970. *The Patient as Person: Explorations in Medical Ethics.* New Haven: Yale University Press, pp. 25, 36, 39.

Ramsey, P. 1978. Ethical dimensions of experimental research on children. In *Research on Children: Medical Imperatives, Ethical Quandaries.* Jan Van Eys, ed. Baltimore: University Park Press. Pp. 61–67.

Reiss, T. F., L. C. Altman, P. Chervinsky, A. Bewtram. W. E. Stricker, G. P. Noonan, S. Kundu, and J. Zha. 1996. Effects of montelukast (MK-0476), a new potent cysteinyl leukotriene (LTD4) receptor antagonist, in patients with chronic asthma. *Journal of Allergy and Clinical Immunology* 98:528–534.

Relling, M. V., P. L. Harrison, and W. E. Evans. 1999. Cytochrome P450 in normal vs. adult human liver. *Clinical Pharmacology and Therapeutics* 65:139.

Riva, R., M. Contin, F. Albani, E. Perucca, G. Procaccianti, and A. Baruzzi. 1985. Free concentration of carbamazepine and carbamazepine-10,11-epoxide in children and adults. Influence of age and phenobarbitone co-medication. *Clinical Pharmacokinetics* 10:524–531.

Schuetz, E. G., J. D. Schuetz, W. M. Grogan, A. Naray-Fejes-Toth, G. Fejes-Toth, J. Raucy, P. Guzelian, K. Gionela, and C. O. Watlington. 1992. Expression of cytochrome P450 3A in amphibian, rat and human kidney. *Archives of Biochemistry and Biophysics* 294:206–214.

Schuetz, J. D., D. L. Beach, and P. S. Guzelian. 1994. Selective expression of cytochrome P450 CYP3A mRNAs in embryonic and adult human liver. *Pharmacogenetics* 4:11–20.

Selroos, O., A. Pietinalho, A. B. Lofroos, and H. Riska. 1995. Effect of early vs. late intervention with inhaled corticosteroids in asthma. *Chest* 108:1228–1234.

Shapiro, G., L. Mendelson, M. Kraemer, M. Cruz-Rivera, and K. Walton-Bowen. 1998. Efficacy and safety of budesonide inhalation suspension (Pulmicort Respules) in young children with inhaled steroid-dependent, persistent asthma. *Journal of Allergy and Clinical Immunology* 102:789–796.

Shimada, T., H. Yamazaki, M. Mimura, Y. Inui, and F. P. Guengerich. 1994. Interindividual variations in human liver cytochrome P450 enzymes involved in the oxidation of drugs, carcinogens and toxic chemicals: Studies with liver microsomes of 30 Japanese and 30 Caucasians. *Journal of Pharmacology and Experimental Therapeutics* 270:414–423.

Silverman, M., and S. Pedersen. 1996. Outcome measures in early childhood asthma and other wheezing disorders. *European Respiratory Journal* 9(Suppl. 21):1S–49S.

Silverman, M., and L. Taussig. 1995. Early childhood asthma: What are the questions? *American Journal of Respiratory Critical Care Medicine* 151:S1–S42.

Sonnier, M., and T. Cresteil. 1998. Delayed ontogeny of CYP1A2 in the human liver. *European Journal of Biochemistry* 251:893–898.

Spector, S. L. 1995. Leukotriene inhibitors and antagonists in asthma. *Annals of Allergy, Asthma, and Immunology* 75:463–470, 473–474.

Spector, S. L., L. J. Smith, and M. Glass. 1994. Effects of 6 weeks of therapy with oral doses of ICI 204,219, a leukotriene D4 receptor antagonist, in subjects with bronchial asthma. *American Journal of Respiratory Critical Care Medicine* 150:618–625.

Tamaoki, J., M. Kondo, N. Sakai, et al. 1997. Leukotriene antagonist prevents exacerbation of asthma during reduction of high-dose inhaled corticosteroid. The Tokyo Joshi-Idai Asthma Research Group. *American Journal of Respiratory Critical Care Medicine* 155:1235–1240.

Tateishi, T., M. Asoh, A. Yamaguchi, T. Yoda, Y. J. Okana, Y. Koitabashi, and S. Kobayashi. 1999. Developmental changes in urinary elimination of theophylline and its metabolites in pediatric patients. *Pediatric Research* 45:66–70.

Thomas, J. K., A. Forrest, S. M. Bhavnani, J. M. Hyatt, A. Cheng, C. H. Ballow, and J. J. Schentag. 1998. Pharmacodynamic evaluation of factors associated with the development of bacterial resistance in acutely ill patients during therapy. *Antimicrobial Agents and Chemotherapy* 42:521–527.

Thummel, K. E., D. O'Shea, M. F. Paine, and D. D. Sheng, K.L. Kunze, J.D. Perkins, and G. Wilkomen. 1996. Oral first-pass elimination of midazolam involves both gastrointestinal and hepatic CYP3A-mediated metabolism. *Clinical Pharmacology and Therapeutics* 59:491–502.

Tjia, J. F., J. Colbert, and D. J. Back. 1996. Theophylline metabolism in human liver microsomes: inhibition studies. *Journal of Pharmacology and Experimental Therapeutics* 276:912–917.

Tran, J. Q., C. H. Ballow, A. Forrest, J. M. Hyatt, M. F. Sands, C. A. Peloquin, and J. J. Schentag. 2000. Comparison of the abilities of grepafloxacin and clarithromycin to eradicate potential bacterial pathogens from the sputa of patients with chronic bronchitis: Influence of pharmacokinetic and pharmacodynamic variables. *Journal of Antimicrobial Chemotherapy* 45:9–17.

Transon, C., S. Lecoeur, T. Leemann, P. Beaune, and P. Dayer. 1996. Interindividual variability in catalytic activity and immunoreactivity of three major human liver cytochrome P450 isozymes. *European Journal of Clinical Pharmacology* 51:79–85.

Treluyer, J. M., G. Chéron, M. Sonnier, and T. Cresteil. 1996. Sudden infant death syndrome and hepatic cytochrome P450 content. *Biochemistry and Pharmacology* 52:497–504.

Treluyer, J. M., G. Gueret, G. Cheron, M. Sonnier, and T. Cresteil. 1997. Developmental expression of CYP2C and CYP2C-dependent activities in the human liver: in vivo/in vitro correlation and inducibility. *Pharmacogenetics* 7:441–452.

Treluyer, J. M., E. Jacqz-Aigrain, F. Alvarez, and T. Cresteil. 1991. Expression of CYP2D6 in the developing human liver. *European Journal of Biochemistry* 202:583–588.

Vieira, I., M. Pasanen, H. Raunio, and T. Cresteil. 1998. Expression of CYP2E1 in human lung and kidney during development and in full term placenta: A differential methylation of the gene is involved in the regulation process. *Pharmacology and Toxicology* 83:183–187.

Vieira, I., M. Sonnier, and T. Cresteil. 1996. Developmental expression of CYP2E1 in the human liver: Hypermethylation control of gene expression during the neonatal period. *European Journal of Biochemistry* 238:476–483.

Wandstrat, T. L., T. J. Schroeder, and S. A. Myre. 1989. Cyclosporine pharmacokinetics in pediatric transplant recipients. *Therapeutic Drug Monitor* 11:493–496.

Watchko, J. F., M. J. Daood, and T. W. Hansen. 1998. Brain bilirubin content is increased in P-glycoprotein-deficient transgenic null mutant mice. *Pediatric Research* 44(5):763–766.

Watkins, P. B. 1994. Noninvasive tests of CYP3A enzymes. *Pharmacogenetics* 4:171–184.

Weiss, S. T. 1995. Early life predictors of adult chronic obstructive lung disease. *European Respiratory Review* 5(31):303–309.

Weithorn, L. A. and S. B. Campbell. 1982. The competency of children and adolescents to make informed treatment decisions. *Child Development* 53(6):1589–1598.

Wenzel, S. E., S. J. Szefler, D. Y. M. Leung, S. I. Sloan, M. D. Rex, and R. J. Martin. 1997. Bronchoscopic evaluation of severe asthma: Persistent inflammation despite high dose glucocorticoids. *American Journal of Respiratory Critical Care Medicine* 156:737–743.

Williams, P. C. 1996. Ethical principles in federal regulations: The case of children and research risks. *Journal of Medicine and Philosophy* 21(2):177–183.

Wilson, J. T., R. D. Brown, J. A. Bocchini, and G. L. Kearns. 1982. Efficacy, disposition and pharmacodynamics of aspirin, acetaminophen and choline salicylate in your febrile children. *Therapeutic Drug Monitor* 4:147.

Wilson, J. T., B. Hojer, and A. Rane. 1976. Loading and conventional dose therapy with phenytoin in children: Kinetic profile of parent drug and main metabolite in plasma. *Clinical Pharmacology and Therapeutics* 20:48–58.

Wilson, J. T., B. Hojer, G. Thompson, A. Rane, and F. Sjoqvist. 1978. High incidence of a concentration dependent skin reaction in children treated with phenytoin. *British Medical Journal* 1(6127):1583.

Woolcock, A. J., and P. J. Barnes. 1996. Asthma: The important questions. Part 3. *American Journal of Respiratory Critical Care Medicine* 153(Suppl.):S1–S32.

Yaffe, S. J., A. Rane, F. Sjoqvist, L. O. Boreus, and S. Orrenius. 1970. The presence of a monooxygenase system in human fetal liver microsomes. *Life Science* 9:1189–1200.

A

Workshop Agenda

ROUNDTABLE ON RESEARCH AND DEVELOPMENT OF DRUGS, BIOLOGICS, AND MEDICAL DEVICES

Rational Therapeutics for Infants and Children

24–25 May 1999

MONDAY, MAY 24, 1999

Opening Plenary

8:30 a.m. **Welcome and Opening Remarks**
Kenneth I. Shine, M.D., President,
Institute of Medicine

8:45 **Statement of Objectives, Charge to Participants, Introductions**
Ronald W. Estabrook, Ph.D., Roundtable Chair,
Virginia Lazenby O'Hara Professor of Biochemistry,
University of Texas Southwestern Medical Center

SESSION I: Similarities and Dissimilarities in Physiology, Metabolism, and Disease States and Responses to Therapy Among Children and Adults

Presentations in this session will address the uniqueness of children and how they are similar or dissimilar to adults with regard to physiology, drug metabolism, immunology, cognitive effects, and response to disease states and therapy. This session will provide the scientific underpinning for the subsequent sessions.

Moderator: Sumner Yaffe, M.D., Roundtable Member,
Director, Center for Research for Mothers and Children,
National Institute for Child Health and Human Development,
National Institutes of Health

9:00 **Characteristics of Infants and Children Versus Adults**
Ralph Kauffman, M.D., Director of Medical Research
Children's Mercy Hospital

9:30 **Differential Drug Response of Children**
John T. Wilson, M.D., Professor and Chief of Clinical
Pharmacology, Department of Pediatrics, Louisiana State
University Medical Center

10:00 **Break**

10:30 **Molecular Basis of Drug Metabolism**
Thierry Cresteil, Ph.D., Director of Research,
Centre National de la Recherche Scientifique,
Institut Gustave Roussy, Villejuif, France

11:00 **Gene Expression-Ontogeny of Drug Metabolism**
Steve Leeder, Pharm.D., Ph.D., Associate Professor of
Pediatrics and Pharmacology, Children's Mercy Hospital

Special Address
11:30 **Science, Challenges, and Children**
Jane Henney, M.D., Commissioner,
U.S. Food and Drug Administration

12:15 p.m. **Lunch Break**

SESSION II: Pharmacokinetics and Pharmacodynamics in Children Versus Adults

Presentations in Session II will identify new advances in biomedical science that are uniquely applicable to children and that could be applied to the development and testing of drugs and biologics for children.

Moderator: Whaijen Soo, M.D., Ph.D., Roundtable Member,
Vice President, Clinical Services
Roche Pharmaceuticals, Hoffmann-La Roche, Inc.

1:30 p.m.	**Drug Metabolism in Children and Adolescents: Insights from Therapeutic Adventures** Greg Kearns, Pharm.D., Professor of Pediatrics, Pharmacology and Therapeutics, and Chief, Division of Pediatric Clinical Pharmacology, Children's Mercy Hospital
2:00	**Ontogeny of P-Glycoprotein as a Transporter** John Watchko, M.D., Associate Professor of Pediatrics, Obstetrics, Gynecology, and Reproductive Science, University of Pittsburgh School of Medicine, and Department of Pediatrics, Magee Women's Hospital
2:30	**Glucose Transporters-Developmental Aspects** Sherin U. Devaskar, M.D., Professor of Pediatrics, Obstetrics, Gynecology, and Reproductive Science, University of Pittsburgh School of Medicine, and Chief of Pediatrics, Magee Women's Hospital
3:00	**Formulations** Emmett Clemente, Ph.D., Chairman and Founder, Ascent Pediatrics, Inc.
3:30	**Break**
3:45	**Anti-Infectives** Charles H. Ballow, Pharm.D., Director, Anti-Infective Research, Kaleida Health Millard Fillmore Hospital
4:15	**Rational Therapeutics for Childhood Asthma** Stanley J. Szefler, M.D., Helen Wohlberg and Henry Lambert Chair in Pharmacokinetics, Director of Clinical Pharmacology, National Jewish Medical and Research Center, and Professor of Pediatrics, and Pharmacology, University of Colorado Health Sciences Center
4:45	**Oncology** David Poplack, M.D., Elise C. Young Professor of Pediatric Oncology, and Head, Hematology Oncology Section, Department of Pediatrics Baylor College of Medicine and Texas Children's Cancer Center
5:15	**Adjournment and Reception in the Great Hall for Roundtable Members, Participants, and Guests**

TUESDAY, MAY 25, 1999

8:00 a.m. **Opening Remarks**
Ronald Estabrook, Ph.D., Roundtable Chair

SESSION III: Extrapolation of Safety and Efficacy Data for Children

This session will examine the special requirements in evaluating drugs and biologics in pediatric populations. Questions to be explored include when and how safety and efficacy data can be used for children.

Moderator: Michael R. McGarvey, M.D., Roundtable Member, Chief Medical Officer, Blue Cross and Blue Shield of New Jersey, Inc.

8:15 **Special Considerations for Evaluating Medical Devices in Infants and Children**
David Feigal, Jr, M.D., Director [Designate], Center for Devices and Radiological Health, U.S. Food and Drug Administration

8:45 **Defining Surrogate Endpoints and Biomarkers for Drug Action in Pediatric Trials**
Robert Temple, M.D., Associate Director for Medical Policy, Center for Drug Evaluation and Research, U.S. Food and Drug Administration

9:15 **Prediction of Long-Term Effects on Postnatal Brain Development**
Mark Batshaw, M.D., Chair of Pediatrics, George Washington University Medical Center, and Director, Children's Research Institute, Children's National Medical Center

9:45 **Evaluating Biological Therapeutics in Pediatric Clinical Trials**
Karen Weiss, M.D., Director, Division of Clinical Trial Design and Analysis, Center for Biologics Evaluation and Research, U.S. Food and Drug Administration

10:15 **Break**

APPENDIX A

SESSION IV: Raising Awareness of Regulatory, Legal, and Ethical Issues

This session will examine the many interrelated legal and regulatory issues in evaluating new drugs and biologics for pediatric populations. The session will also examine the interrelated social and ethical concerns when evaluating drugs and biologics with children.

Moderator: The Honorable Paul G. Rogers, J.D., Roundtable Member, Partner, Hogan & Hartson, Former Member, U.S. House of Representatives

10:30 **FDA Perspective on New Regulations**
Dianne Murphy, M.D., Associate Director for Pediatrics, Center for Drug Evaluation and Research, U.S. Food and Drug Administration

11:00 **The Role of IRB and Data Safety Boards**
Susan Ellenberg, Ph.D., Division of Biostatistics and Epidemiology, Center for Biologics Evaluation and Research, U.S. Food and Drug Administration

11:30 **Ethics of Drug and Biologic Research in Infants and Children**
Robert M. ("Skip") Nelson, M.D., Ph.D., Associate Professor of Pediatrics and Bioethics, Medical College of Wisconsin

12:00 noon **Legal and Regulatory Considerations for the Conduct of Pediatric Clinical Trials**
Michael Labson, J.D., Covington & Burling

12:30 p.m. **International Pediatric Drug Development: An Industry Perspective**
Steven Spielberg, M.D., Global Head, Pediatric Drug Development, R.W. Johnson Pharmaceutical Research Institute

1:00 **Lunch Break**

2:00 **Panel Discussion**
Panelists:
Susan Ellenberg, Ph.D,
Michael Labson, J.D.

　　　　　　Michael R. McGarvey, M.D.
　　　　　　Dianne Murphy, M.D.
　　　　　　Robert M. Nelson, M.D., Ph.D.,
　　　　　　The Honorable Paul G. Rogers, J.D.
　　　　　　Steven Spielberg, M.D.
　　　　　　Sumner Yaffe, M.D.

3:00　　**Conclusions**
　　　　　　Murray Lumpkin, M.D., Deputy Director for Review
　　　　　　Management, Center for Drug Evaluation and Research,
　　　　　　U.S. Food and Drug Administration

3:30　　**Closing Remarks**
　　　　　　Ronald Estabrook, Ph.D., Roundtable Chair

4:45　　**Adjournment**

B

Biographies

ROUNDTABLE MEMBERS

RONALD W. ESTABROOK, Ph.D. (*Chair*), graduated with a B.S. from Rensselaer Polytechnic Institute, Troy, New York. Dr. Estabrook did his graduate training in biochemistry at the University of Rochester, Rochester, N.Y. (Ph.D. 1954). He then accepted a postdoctoral position in biophysics to work with Britton Chance at the Johnson Research Foundation, University of Pennsylvania. In 1959, Dr. Estabrook joined the faculty of the School of Medicine of the University of Pennsylvania where he advanced to the rank of professor of physical biochemistry. It was during this time, in the early 1960s, that Dr. Estabrook, together with Drs. David Cooper and Otto Rosenthal of the Department of Surgery of the University of Pennsylvania, carried out studies in which they discovered the enzymatic (functional) properties of the heme protein, now known as cytochrome P450. In 1968, Dr. Estabrook moved to Dallas, Texas, to serve as Virginia Lazenby O'Hara Professor of Biochemistry and Chairman of the Department of Biochemistry at the University of Texas Southwestern Medical School. He served as the first Dean of the Graduate School of Biomedical Sciences at the Dallas campus of the University of Texas. Dr. Estabrook has coauthored more than 260 publications and has edited 14 books. He has received many honors including election to the National Academy of Sciences in 1979 and the awarding of an honorary Doctor of Medicine from the Karolinska Institut in Stockholm, Sweden, in 1981, and a Doctor of Science from the University of Rochester, also in 1981.

ARTHUR L. BEAUDET, M.D., is an investigator at the Howard Hughes Medical Institute. Dr. Beaudet is also the Henry and Emma Meyer Professor of

Molecular and Human Genetics and acting chair of that department at the Baylor College of Medicine in Texas.

LESLIE Z. BENET, Ph.D., is Professor and former Chairman (1978–1998), Department of Biopharmaceutical Sciences, University of California, San Francisco, and Chairman of the Board, AvMax, Inc. He received his A.B. in English, B.S. in pharmacy, and M.S. from the University of Michigan and Ph.D. from the University of California. He has received five honorary doctorates: Uppsala University, Uppsala, Sweden (Pharm.D., 1987); Leiden University, Leiden, The Netherlands (Ph.D., 1995); University of Illinois at Chicago (D.Sc., 1997); Philadelphia College of Pharmacy and Science (D.Sc., 1997); and Long Island University (D.Sc., 1999). His research interests and more than 390 publications are in the areas of pharmacokinetics, biopharmaceutics, and pharmacodynamics. He is a Fellow of the Academy of Pharmaceutical Sciences, the American Association of Pharmaceutical Scientists, and of the American Association for the Advancement of Science (AAAS). In 1982, Dr. Benet received the American Pharmaceutical Association's Academy of Pharmaceutical Sciences Research Achievement Award in Pharmaceutics and the University of Michigan's College of Pharmacy Distinguished Alumnus Award. In 1985, he served as President of the Academy of Pharmaceutical Sciences. In 1987, Dr. Benet was elected to membership in the Institute of Medicine of the National Academies. He presently serves as Chair of the U.S. Food and Drug Administration's Expert Panel on Individual Bioequivalence and Chair of the Board of Pharmaceutical Sciences of the International Pharmaceutical Federation, and the Board of Directors of the American Foundation for Pharmaceutical Education. He is a board member, scientific board member, or consultant for more than 20 pharmaceutical and biotechnology companies and Treasurer for the International Society for the Study of Xenobiotics. Dr. Benet is the editor of several medical and scientific books.

D. BRUCE BURLINGTON, M.D. (ex officio), is Director of the Center for Devices and Radiological Health at the U.S. Food and Drug Administration (FDA). He was formerly Deputy Director of the Office of Drug Evaluation II in the Center of Drug Evaluation and Research. Dr. Burlington served as Acting Director of the Office of Generic Drugs for 1 year and served as Deputy Director for Medical Affairs of the Center for almost 2 years. In his medical affairs position, he was active in jurisdictional issues, international harmonization of drug approval standards, the planning and implementation of user fees, accountability of program actions on clinical holds and refusal to file, and the effective use of FDA's scientific advisory committees.

ROBERT M. CALIFF, M.D., is Associate Vice Chancellor for Clinical Research, Committee on Health Information Policy and Services, and chief executive officer of the Duke Clinical Research Institute. He graduated from Duke University summa cum laude and Phi Beta Kappa in 1973 and from Duke University Medical School in 1978, where he was selected for Alpha Omega Alpha. He is a certified specialist in internal medicine (1984) and cardiovascular disease (1986) and a Fellow of the American College of Cardiology (1988). He did his internship and residency at the University of California, San Francisco, and a fellowship in cardiology at Duke University. He is currently Associate Vice Chancellor for Clinical Research, Director of the Duke Clinical Research Institute, and Professor of Medicine, Division of Cardiology, at the Duke University Medical Center, Durham, North Carolina. He is also editor of the *American Heart Journal*. Dr. Califf has led the Coordinating Center effort for many of the best-known cardiology trials of recent years, including CAVEAT (Coronary Angioplasty Versus Excisional Atherectomy Trial), GUSTO (Global Utilization of Streptokinases and t-PA for Occluded Coronary Arteries), EPIC (Evaluation of c7E3 Fab in Preventing Ischemic Complications of High-Risk Angioplasty), and TAMI (Thrombolysis and Angioplasty in Myocardial Infarction). In conjunction with colleagues at the Duke Databank for Cardiovascular Disease, he has written extensively about clinical and economic outcomes in chronic ischecon heart disease. He is editor of *Acute Coronary Care*, second edition. He is a section editor in the *Textbook of Cardiovascular Medicine* and is the author of more than 500 peer-reviewed articles.

MICHAEL D. CLAYMAN, M.D., is Vice President of Cardiovascular Research and Decision Phase Medical for Lilly Research Laboratories, a division of Eli Lilly & Company. He had been Vice President of Product Development and Technology for Advanced Cardiovascular Systems, Inc., a subsidiary of Eli Lilly & Company located in Santa Clara, California, since 1992. He received a Bachelor of Arts degree, cum laude, in molecular biophysics and biochemistry from Yale University in 1974. In 1978 he was awarded a doctor of medicine degree from the University of California at San Diego School of Medicine. Following completion of his internship and residency in internal medicine at the Herbert C. Moffitt University of California Hospitals at San Francisco in 1981, Dr. Clayman completed clinical and research fellowships in nephrology at the University of Pennsylvania. He is recipient of the Physician Scientist Award from the National Institutes of Health. Dr. Clayman joined Lilly in 1987 as an associate clinical research physician. He was named clinical research physician in 1989. In 1990, he became Director of the Internal Medicine Division and later that year became Director of Clinical Pharmacology at the Lilly Clinic, serving in that capacity until 1992. He is a member of the American Society of Nephrology, the American Federation for Clinical Research, the American Association of Immunologists, and the American Heart Association.

ADRIAN L. EDWARDS, M.D., is a retired private practice cardiologist in New York State. Dr. Edwards received his bachelor's degree from Wagner College in New York and his medical degree from Howard University in Washington, D.C. Previously, Dr. Edwards was Clinical Assistant Professor of Medicine at Cornell University Medical College. He was a diplomat for the American Board of Internal Medicine and a fellow for the American College of Physicians. He is a former fellow in cardiology at the New York Hospital, member of the National Medical Association, and a past member of the Board of Governors of St. Barnabas Hospital in the Bronx. Dr. Edwards also served on the Institute of Medicine's Committee on Enhancing the Practice of Occupational and Environmental Medicine.

DAVID W. FEIGAL, JR., M.D., M.P.H. (ex officio), is Director, Center for Devices and Radiological Health, U.S. Food and Drug Administration (FDA). He received his B.S. from the University of Minnesota, M.D. from Stanford University Medical School, and M.P.H. from the University of California at Davis Medical Center, where he remained as Chief Resident and later Residency Program Coordinator before entering a fellowship program in Clinical Epidemiology at the University of California at San Francisco (UCSF). He joined the UCSF faculty in 1984 with joint appointments in the School of Medicine and School of Dentistry as a member of the Department of Medicine and of the Department of Epidemiology and Biostatistics. His academic research interests included clinical epidemiology and clinical trials methodology, in particular, in the therapy of hypertension and AIDS. He came to the FDA in 1992 to head the Division of Anti-Viral Drug Products, a position held until 1997. In 1996, he was also the acting Division Director of the Anti-Infective Drug Division. From 1994 to 1997, he was the Director of the Office of Drug Evaluation IV. In the fall of 1997, he moved to the Center for Biologics Evaluation and Research (CBER) as the Medical Deputy Director. He also served as the CBER ombudsman and had responsibility for the Center's advisory committees. He has been a member of a number of committees and panels sponsored by the World Health Organization, National Institutes of Health, Institute of Medicine, and Centers for Disease Control and Prevention. He has represented FDA at the International Conference on Harmonization, the Tripartite Meetings, and many regulatory meetings.

STEPHEN GROFT, Pharm.D. (ex officio), began his pharmacy career with the Public Health Service in 1970. Stationed first in Chamberlain, South Dakota, and later in Pawnee, Oklahoma, he was responsible for providing pharmacy services to the Indian Health Services Clinics and Hospital in these two service unit areas. In 1974, Dr. Groft transferred to the U.S. Food and Drug Administration (FDA) and served as Executive Secretary to the Psychopharmacologic Agents and the Neurologic Drugs Advisory Committees. Upon receiving his

Pharm.D. degree in 1979 from Duquesne University in Pittsburgh, Pennsylvania, Dr. Groft became involved in FDA's efforts to initiate the Patient Package Insert Program for the labeling of drug products. In 1982, he joined Dr. Marion Finkel in FDA's Office of Orphan Products Development, where his primary area of responsibility was to review those orphan products potentially useful in the treatment of neurologic and psychiatric disorders. Dr. Groft was the Executive Secretary of the U.S. Department of Health and Human Services' Orphan Products Board from 1982 to 1986, and until 1989 coordinated the activities of the National Commission on Orphan Diseases as the Executive Director. When the Office of Rare Diseases was formally created at the National Institutes of Health in 1993, Dr. Groft was selected as its Director. He also served as the first Acting Director of the National Institutes of Health's Office of Alternative Medicine from 1991 to 1992.

ANNE B. JACKSON, M.A., R.N., recently completed her second term on the Physician Payment Review Commission. She is a member of the National Legislative Council for the American Association of Retired Persons and has served as chair of the Education Advocacy and Community Service Advisory Committee and as minority spokesperson. Ms. Jackson retired as Professor of Nursing at City University of New York, and has also served as a consumer representative for the Joint Commission on Accreditation of Healthcare Organizations. Ms. Jackson is also a member of the Institute of Medicine Committee on Health Outcomes for Older People.

ROBERT I. LEVY, M.D., joined American Home Products Corporation in 1992 as President of Wyeth-Ayerst Research. On March 6, 1998, he was appointed Senior Vice President, Science and Technology, American Home Products. Before joining American Home Products Corporation, Dr. Levy served as President of The Sandoz Research Institute from 1988 to 1992. Before that he had a distinguished career in research and research management in both government and academia. He was Vice President for Health Sciences and Professor of Medicine at the Columbia University College of Physicians and Surgeons and Vice President and Dean of Tufts University School of Medicine. Dr. Levy also served at the National Institutes of Health (NIH), with the last 6 years as Director of the National Heart, Lung, and Blood Institute. His 18-year tenure at NIH included pathfinding work in the areas of cholesterol, lipids, lipoproteins, atherosclerosis, and heart disease. Dr. Levy is a graduate of Cornell University and Yale University School of Medicine, cum laude. He is a member of numerous honorary and professional societies including Phi Beta Kappa, Alpha Omega Alpha, and the American College of Cardiology. He is also a member of the Institute of Medicine of the National Academy of Sciences. He also serves as chairman of the Pharmaceuticals Research and Manufacturers of America Science and Regulatory Section Executive Committee. Dr. Levy is the author or coauthor of more than 300 scientific publications.

MICHAEL R. McGARVEY, M.D., is Chief Medical Officer for Horizon Blue Cross Blue Shield of New Jersey. As Chief Medical Officer, Dr. McGarvey is responsible for medical policy development and application, health care data analysis and cost management activities, and clinical quality improvement work. Dr. McGarvey has more than 25 years of experience in health care delivery and administration. Before joining Horizon Blue Cross Blue Shield of New Jersey he was Managing Director of Health Strategies for the Alexander & Alexander Consulting Group, a leading international human resources and benefits consulting organization. Previously, he was an executive with Empire Blue Cross and Blue Shield, New York, first as Vice President of Health Services Management, and then as Corporate Vice President of Health Affairs. He is a former Chief Medical Officer and Deputy Director for the New York State Department of Health's Office of Health Systems Management and a former Vice President for Health Affairs and Professor of Health Services at Hunter College of the City University of New York. Dr. McGarvey is a member of the National Council on Medical Management of the Blue Cross and Blue Shield Association, a former trustee of the New York Academy of Medicine, and former chairman of the New York Statewide Cardiac Advisory Committee. Dr. McGarvey received his medical degree from the University of Southern California School of Medicine and his bachelor's degree from Reed College.

KSHITIJ MOHAN, Ph.D., is a Corporate Vice President for Baxter International Inc. He is responsible for corporate research and technical services, including research centers in the United States and Europe, as well as emerging technology ventures and technology strategy development. He is also the founder and leader of the Baxter Technical Council, which includes Baxter's technical leaders from around the world, and he serves on the Baxter Operating Management Team. Dr. Mohan joined Baxter in 1988. Before joining Baxter, Dr. Mohan served in various capacities in the U.S. Food and Drug Administration (FDA). Between 1979 and 1983, Dr. Mohan served in the White House Office of Management and Budget with responsibilities for national research and development (R&D) policies, programs of the National Science Foundation, and the National Aeronautic and Space Administration's Aeronautical and Space Research and Technology programs. During this time, he also served on two task forces of the White House and led an interagency study of the U.S. Antarctic program. Before 1979, Dr. Mohan was a researcher at the National Bureau of Standards (now the National Institute for Standards and Technology) in the fields of applied optics and superconductivity. He has published widely in the fields of health policies, regulations, research and development policies, and applied physics. He has lectured and consulted extensively in the United States,

Britain, Spain, Brazil, the Philippines, Japan, Australia, and the People's Republic of China. He is the recipient of numerous awards from Baxter, the White House, and U.S. government agencies and civic groups, including FDA's highest award, the Award of Merit, on two occasions. He is a director of the Health Industry Manufacturers' Association and KeraVision, Inc. He is or has been a member of the Baxter Japan Board, the Corporate Advisory Boards of Engineering Schools at Dartmouth College and the University of California, the Review Board of the President Truman Foundation, the Board of Directors of the Regulatory Affairs Professional Society, and various editorial boards. Dr. Mohan earned a Ph.D. in physics from Georgetown University and has received extensive training in management.

STUART L. NIGHTINGALE, M.D. (ex officio), is Associate Commissioner for Health Affairs and Senior Health Adviser, Office of International and Constituent Relations, U.S. Food and Drug Administration (FDA). He received a B.A. degree from Yale University and an M.D. degree from the New York University School of Medicine. He served his internship and residency in internal medicine at Montefiore Hospital and Medical Center in New York. He received additional training in anatomical pathology (Bellevue Hospital) and adolescent medicine (Montefiore Hospital). He served on the faculties of the Johns Hopkins University School of Medicine, and the State University of New York (Downstate) School of Medicine. He worked for the State of Maryland Department of Health and Mental Hygiene and entered federal service at the Special Action Office for Drug Abuse Prevention, Executive Office of the President. Before joining FDA he spent 3 years at the National Institute on Drug Abuse as a division director. At FDA he has held a number of positions in the Bureau of Drugs (predecessor to the Center for Drug Evaluation and Research) and in the Office of the Commissioner that have included responsibility for coordinating FDA's outreach to health professional organizations and outreach to the human subject protection community and for coordinating FDA's international activities, especially its relations with the World Health Organization. He has written extensively on regulatory and health professional matters.

PAUL GRANT ROGERS, J.D., is a partner in the law firm of Hogan & Hartson in Washington, D.C. He was a member of the U.S. Congress from 1955 to 1979 and Chairman of the House of Representatives Subcommittee on Health and the Environment. Some of the prominent pieces of legislation that Mr. Rogers sponsored or played a major role in enacting are National Cancer Act of 1971 and 1977; Health Manpower Training Act; Heart, Lung and Blood Act; Research on Aging Act; Comprehensive Drug Abuse Prevention and Control Act of 1970; Medical Device Amendments of 1976; Emergency Medical Services Act; Health Maintenance Organization Act; Clean Air Act; Safe Drinking Water Act; and the Medicare-Medicaid Anti-Fraud and Abuse Amendments of 1977. Mr. Rogers serves as Chair at Research!America, the National Foundation for Infectious Diseases Board of Trustees, the National Osteoporosis Foundation, and the Friends of the National Library of Medicine. He is Cochair of the National Leadership Coalition on Health Care. Mr. Rogers has received honorary degrees from various universities and has received many distinguished service awards. He is a member of the Harvard School of Public Health Dean's Council, the Board of Trustees of the University of Pennsylvania Medical Center, the Council of the Washington University School of Medicine, the University of Chicago Council for the Division of the Biological Sciences and the Pritzker School of Medicine, and the Whitehead Institute Board of Advisors. He is also a member of the Institute of Medicine of the National Academy of Sciences.

DANIEL SECKINGER, M.D., was formerly Group Vice President of Professional Standards at the American Medical Association. His responsibilities included science and technology, medical education, ethics and quality/managed care. Previously, Dr. Seckinger was the President of the College of American Pathologists (CAP). Prior to his election as President of the CAP, Dr. Seckinger served on the Board of Governors for six years and as Chairman of the Council on Scientific Affairs for four years. Dr. Seckinger has practiced in South Florida for the past 30 years. In 1984 he was elected President of the Dade County Medical Association and has also served as President of the American Center Society in South Florida. Dr. Seckinger was formerly Clinical Professor of Pathology at the University of Miami School of Medicine and founder and director of the Oncology Laboratory in his primary practice environment of Cedars Medical Center. Dr. Seckinger has published extensively on tumor markers and DNA ploidy and cell cycle studies in the *Prognosis of Cancer*. For four years he directed the Cancer Program at Cedars, interacting with over 40 medical, surgical, radiological, and gynecological oncologists. Dr. Seckinger received his M.D. from George Washington University in Washington, D.C., in 1954 and served as resident in Pathology for five years and Surgery for three years. He is certified by the American Board of Pathology in Anatomic and Clinical Pathology.

WHAIJEN SOO, M.D., Ph.D., is Vice President, Clinical Sciences, Hoffmann-La Roche Inc. As Vice President of Clinical Sciences at Hoffmann-La Roche Inc., Dr. Soo is responsible for the planning and execution of global development and life cycle management, and of new anticancer drugs and antiviral and immunotherapies against AIDS and other viral diseases, as well as drugs used for transplantation. His groups in Nutley, N.J., Basel, Switzerland, Welwyn, United Kingdom, Mannheim, Germany, and Palo Alto, Calif., also provide clinical expert advice to global research projects at all stages and participate in the transition planning and execution of projects from research to development. In addition, his groups participate in global licensing activities and strategic planning at the therapeutic area level with research and business colleagues. For the United States-based groups, Dr. Soo also has administrative responsibilities for all clinical science groups, including the four clinical science therapeutic clusters covering all therapeutic areas, clinical pharmacology group, and clinical safety surveillance and risk management group. Dr. Soo received a Ph.D. in biochemistry from the University of California, Berkeley. He also has a M.D. from the University of California, San Francisco, and received postgraduate training at Harvard Medical School in Boston. He has extensive experience with drug development in various therapeutic areas including virology, immunology, oncology, nervous systems, and endocrinology and metabolism. Overall, he has either been directly involved or supervised the successful submissions and registration of 14 new drug or biologics applications worldwide.

REED V. TUCKSON, M.D., is Senior Vice President for the American Medical Association (AMA). Dr. Tuckson's areas of responsibility include medical education (undergraduate, graduate, and continuing medical education); ethics; science, technology, and public health; quality and managed care; and the National Patient Safety Foundation. Before joining AMA, Dr. Tuckson was President of the Charles R. Drew University School of Medicine and Science in Los Angeles, California, from 1991 to 1997. From 1986 to 1990, Dr. Tuckson was Commissioner of Public Health for the District of Columbia. From 1990 to 1991, he served as Senior Vice President for Programs at the March of Dimes Birth Defects Foundation. He also serves on a number of health care, academic, and federal boards and committees, and is a nationally known lecturer on topics concerning community-based medicine, the moral responsibilities of health professionals, and physician leadership. Dr. Tuckson is a graduate of the Georgetown University School of Medicine. He completed his internship, residency, and fellowship in general internal medicine at the Hospital of the University of Pennsylvania. During his fellowship, he also became a Robert Wood Johnson Foundation Clinical Scholar at the University of Pennsylvania, where he studied health care administration and health policy at the Wharton School of Business and where he was active in ambulatory, student health, prevention, and geriatric clinical care settings.

JANET WOODCOCK, M.D. (ex officio), is Director of the Center for Drug Evaluation and Research. Before that she was Director of the Office of Therapeutics Research and Review, Center for Biologics Evaluation and Research (CBER) at the U.S. Food and Drug Administration (FDA). Dr. Woodcock is an internist/rheumatologist with research experience in immunology. She joined FDA in 1985. She served as Director of the Division of Biological Investigational New Drugs in CBER from 1988 to 1992 and was Acting Deputy Director of the Center in 1991 and 1992. Dr. Woodcock received her M.D. from Northwestern Medical School and completed further training and held faculty appointment at the Pennsylvania State University and the University of California at San Francisco.

SUMNER YAFFE, M.D. (ex officio), Director of the Center for Research for Mothers and Children at the National Institutes of Health, received his A.B. in chemistry and M.A. in pharmacology from Harvard University and his medical degree from the University of Vermont School of Medicine. Dr. Yaffe's honors include a Fulbright Scholarship; the Lederle Medical Faculty Award, Wall Memorial Lecturer; Editor, *Pediatric Clinics of North America*; Upjohn Lecturer; Louisville Pediatric Lectureship; Guest Editor, *Clinics in Perinatology*; Creasy Visiting Professorship; and the Hardt Memorial Lecturer. He is an honorary member of the Society of Perinatal Obstetricians and a member of the Alpha Omega Alpha and Sigma Xi honorary societies. Dr. Yaffe has held academic and staff appointments at Stanford University Medical Center, State University of New York at Buffalo, Children's Hospital of Buffalo, and at the University of Pennsylvania and Children's Hospital of Philadelphia. Dr. Yaffe has also served as a member or chair of more than 40 committees and advisory boards of organizations dealing with child health and clinical pharmacology. Dr. Yaffe has published more than 200 articles in the area of pediatrics and clinical pharmacology.

KATHRYN ZOON, Ph.D. (ex officio), became Director of the Center for Biologics Evaluation and Research (CBER), U.S. Food and Drug Administration (FDA), in March 1992. Dr. Zoon was formerly the Director of the Division of Cytokine Biology in CBER, where she was actively involved with regulatory issues related to cytokines, growth factors, and studies on interferon purification, characterization, and receptors. Dr. Zoon worked at the National Institutes of Health (NIH) from 1975 to 1980 with Nobel Prize Laureate Christian B. Anfinsen on the production and purification of human interferons. She continued her work on interferons and reviewed cytokine products when she joined FDA in 1980. She received her B.S. degree, cum laude, in chemistry from Rensselear Polytechnic Institute in 1970 and was granted a Ph.D. in biochemistry from The Johns Hopkins University in 1975. Dr. Zoon is an editor of the *Journal of Interferon Research* and the author of numerous scientific papers on interferons. She has received numerous awards, including the NIH Lectureship (1994), Sydney Riegelman Lectureship (1994), Biopharm Person of the Year Award (1992), the *Genetic Engineering News* Award (1994) for streamlining and improving the regulatory process for biologics and biotechnology products, and the Meritorious Executive Rank Award (1994) for sustained superior performance in revitalizing and reorganizing CBER to meet the challenges of new responsibilities and new technologies.

STUDY STAFF

JONATHAN R. DAVIS, Ph.D., is a Senior Program Officer at the Institute of Medicine (IOM). His primary charge is the Study Director of IOM's Forum on Emerging Infections and the Roundtable on Research and Development of Drugs, Biologics, and Medical Devices. Dr. Davis was formerly the Science Officer for the Emerging Infectious Diseases and HIV/AIDS Program in the U.S. Department of State's Bureau of Oceans and International Environmental and Scientific Affairs. Before his work at the State Department, Dr. Davis was an Assistant Professor of Medicine and Head of the Malaria Laboratory at the University of Maryland School of Medicine, where he was the principle and coprinciple investigator on grants investigating the fundamental biology of malaria transmission and on the development and testing of candidate malaria vaccines in human volunteers. Dr. Davis has an M.S. in medical entomology and parasitology from Clemson University and a Ph.D. in immunology and infectious diseases from The Johns Hopkins University School of Hygiene and Public Health. Dr. Davis is an ad hoc reviewer for several professional scientific journals and holds adjunct faculty appointments at The Johns Hopkins University School of Hygiene and Public Health, the University of Maryland School of Medicine, and the Uniformed Services University School of the Health Sciences.

PETER BOUXSEIN, J.D., is a Senior Program Officer in the Institute of Medicine. Mr. Bouxsein has an undergraduate degree in science from Carnegie Mellon University and a law degree from the University of Chicago. He has 23 years of service with the federal government, including the U.S. Department of Justice, the Office of Economic Opportunity, the Health Care Financing Administration, and the Agency for Health Care Policy and Research, in the areas of civil rights, higher education, and health care. Seven of those years were spent as counsel to the Subcommittee on Health and the Environment, U.S. House of Representatives, focusing on Medicare, health care technology, graduate medical education, and clinical research. In addition, Mr. Bouxsein has served as the Deputy Director of the Institute for Public Policy Studies, University of Michigan, and Deputy Executive Vice President of the American College of Physicians. He is also a research associate and lecturer at the Johns Hopkins School of Public Health.

SARAH PITLUCK, M.S., is a research assistant in the Division of Health Sciences Policy at the Institute of Medicine (IOM). Sarah helps support the IOM's Committee on Understanding the Biology of Sex and Gender Differences and the Roundtable on Environmental Health Sciences, Research, and Medicine. She also assists the Forum on Emerging Infections and the Roundtable on Research and Development of Drugs, Biologics, and Medical Devices. She received her undergraduate degree in political science at Washington University in St. Louis, Missouri, before completing her master's degree in public policy and public administration at the London School of Economics and Political Science.

Sarah's master's thesis addresses the sources of divergent policies toward screening for prostate cancer in the United States and United Kingdom. Sarah's most recent IOM publications include *Fluid Resuscitation: State of the Science for Treating Combat Casualties and Civilian Injuries* and *Organ Procurement and Transplantation Policy: Assessing Current Policies and the Potential Impact of the DHHS Final Rule.*

VIVIAN P. NOLAN, M.A., is the Research Associate for the Forum on Emerging Infections and for the Roundtable on Research and Development of Drugs, Biologics, and Medical Devices. Before joining the Institute of Medicine, Ms. Nolan was a science assistant in the Division of Environmental Biology at the National Science Foundation (NSF) where she worked on grants administration, research projects, and policy analyses on environmental and conservation biology issues. Ms. Nolan is a recipient of an NSF Directors Award for the policy-oriented, interdisciplinary Water and Watersheds collaborative NSF/Envir-onmental Protection Agency grants program. Ms. Nolan is pursuing her doctorate degree in environmental science and public policy from George Mason University. Her graduate work has included research and policy analysis on such issues as environmental, biodiversity conservation, sustainable development, human health, and emerging and reemerging infectious diseases. In August 1998, she participated in an educational program in Kenya where she studied the relationship between ecological degradation and emerging infectious diseases. Ms. Nolan was awarded an M.A. in science, technology, and public policy in 1994 from the George Washington University, and in 1987, she simultaneously earned two bachelor's degrees in international studies and Latin American studies.

NICOLE AMADO was the Project Assistant for the Forum on Emerging Infections, as well as for the Roundtable on Research and Development of Drugs, Biologics, and Medical Devices. Ms. Amado was formerly a Project Coordinator for the Cystic Fibrosis Foundation. Before her work at the Cystic Fibrosis Foundation, she was a Panel Assistant with the Chemical Manufacturers Association. Ms. Amado brings to the Institute of Medicine considerable experience in project organization, research and analysis, and administrative problem solving. Ms. Amado earned a bachelor's degree in biology from the University of Louisville in 1994.